Practising Evidence-based
PRIMARY CARE

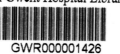
Tim Lancaster

Department of Primary Care
Institute of Health Sciences
Old Road, Headington
Oxford OX3 7LF

Editor
Sharon Straus

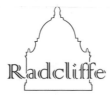

Radcliffe

Radcliffe Medical Press
18 Marcham Road, Abingdon, Oxon OX14 1AA, UK
Tel: 01235 528820 Fax: 01235 528830
e-mail: medical@radpress.win-uk.net

Radcliffe Medical Press Ltd
18 Marcham Road, Abingdon, Oxon OX14 1AA

British Library Cataloguing in Publication Data

A catalogue record for this book is available from the British Library.

ISBN 1 85775 405 0

Typeset by Advance Typesetting Ltd, Oxfordshire
Printed and bound by Hobbs the Printers, Totton, Hampshire

SESSION	TOPIC

CONTENTS

ACKNOWLEDGEMENTS

Radcliffe Medical Press acknowledges with gratitude the kind permission granted by publishers of the citation references for the full papers to be reproduced at the beginning of each session. These permissions prohibit further reproduction by photocopying or by electronic means and if this facility is required, further permission should be obtained from the source quoted in each case.

Extracts from *Evidence-based Medicine: how to practice and teach EBM* (David Sackett *et al.*) which appear at the back of this manual are reproduced with the kind permission of Harcourt Brace & Co Ltd.

This is a syllabus for a 7 session course for those working in primary care to practise evidence-based medicine: that is, how to integrate our individual clinical expertise and knowledge of individual patients with a critical appraisal of the best available external clinical evidence from systematic research. This manual is one of a series in different clinical areas. The problems and examples are selected to be relevant for GPs, GP registrars and medical students. The format and supporting materials are the same as those used in other topic areas, such as general medicine, obstetrics and psychiatry.

We see the practice of evidence-based medicine as a process of life-long, self-directed, problem-based learning in which caring for one's own patients creates the need for clinically important information about diagnosis, prognosis, therapy, and other clinical and healthcare issues, in which its practitioners:

1 convert these information needs into answerable questions;

2 track down, with maximum efficiency, the best evidence with which to answer them (making best use of the increasing variety of sources of primary and secondary evidence);

3 critically appraise that evidence for its validity (closeness to the truth), importance (size of effect) and usefulness (clinical applicability);

4 integrate the appraisal with clinical expertise and apply the results in clinical practice; and

5 evaluate their own performance.

This syllabus is designed to help clinicians develop and improve those skills. In addition, it is designed to help Membership candidates prepare for the EBM portions of the Membership Examination. Ideally, this syllabus should be followed in a group led by a tutor experienced in teaching EBM. However, the manual contains both supporting materials that could allow it to be used for self-study.

Each of its 7 sessions is divided into 2 parts:

Part A: Going through the 5 steps with a patient or practice problem, focusing on step 3 (critical appraisal), step 4 (integration with clinical expertise), and step 5 (self-evaluation). In each example, we present a clinical problem and the evidence which we tracked down to solve it.

You are provided with a worksheet to guide you through the critical appraisal and application of this evidence. In addition, we provide our own completed worksheets for each topic. We hope that the data in these worksheets are accurate, but please understand that the interpretations we offer reflect our own views and biases – you are free to disagree! The explanations given in the worksheets are brief, and you should consult the book *Evidence-based Medicine* for full discussion of the issues – relevant excerpts are included at the end of this manual.

Part B: Skills training, focusing on step 1 (forming answerable clinical questions) and step 2 (finding the best evidence), in which we introduce a variety of sources of evidence plus some strategies for analysing, summarising and storing the evidence in the form of one-page summaries ('Critically Appraised Topics' or CATs).

Evidence-based Medicine: what it is and what it isn't

This is the text of an editorial from the *British Medical Journal* of 13th January 1996 (*BMJ* 1996; **312**: 71–2)

Authors:

David L Sackett, Professor, NHS Research and Development Centre for Evidence-based Medicine, Oxford.

William MC Rosenberg, Clinical Tutor in Medicine, Nuffield Department of Clinical Medicine, Oxford.

JA Muir Gray, Director of Research and Development, Anglia and Oxford Regional Health Authority, Milton Keynes.

R Brian Haynes, Professor of Medicine and Clinical Epidemiology, McMaster University Hamilton, Canada.

W Scott Richardson, Rochester, USA.

Evidence-based medicine, whose philosophical origins extend back to mid-19th century Paris and earlier, remains a hot topic for clinicians, public health practitioners, purchasers, planners and the public. There are now frequent workshops in how to practice and teach it (one sponsored by this journal will be held in London on April 24th); undergraduate [1] and post-graduate training programmes [2] are incorporating it [3] (or pondering how to do so); British centres for evidence-based practice have been established or planned in adult medicine, child health, surgery, pathology, pharmacotherapy, nursing, general practice, and dentistry; the Cochrane Collaboration and the York Centre for Review and Dissemination in York are providing systematic reviews of the effects of health care; new evidence-based practice journals are being launched; and it has become a common topic in the lay media. But enthusiasm has been mixed with some negative reaction [4–6]. Criticism has ranged from evidence-based medicine being old-hat to it being a dangerous innovation, perpetrated by the arrogant to serve cost-cutters and suppress clinical freedom. As evidence-based medicine continues to evolve and adapt, now is a useful time to refine the discussion of what it is and what it is not.

Evidence-based medicine is the conscientious, explicit and judicious use of current best evidence in making decisions about the care of individual patients. The practice of evidence-based medicine means integrating individual clinical expertise with the best available external clinical evidence from systematic research. By individual clinical expertise we mean the proficiency and judgement that individual clinicians acquire through clinical experience and clinical practice. Increased expertise is reflected in many ways, but especially in more effective and efficient diagnosis and in the more thoughtful identification and compassionate use of individual patients' predicaments, rights, and preferences in making clinical decisions about their care. By best available external clinical evidence we mean clinically relevant research, often from the basic sciences of medicine, but especially from patient centred clinical research into the accuracy and precision of diagnostic tests (including the clinical examination), the power of prognostic markers, and the efficacy and safety of therapeutic, rehabilitative, and preventive regimens. External clinical evidence both invalidates previously accepted diagnostic tests and treatments and replaces them with new ones that are more powerful, more accurate, more efficacious, and safer.

Good doctors use both individual clinical expertise and the best available external evidence, and neither alone is enough. Without clinical expertise, practice risks becoming tyrannised by evidence, for even excellent external evidence may be inapplicable to or inappropriate for an individual patient. Without current best evidence, practice risks becoming rapidly out of date, to the detriment of patients.

This description of what evidence-based medicine is helps clarify what evidence-based medicine is not. Evidence-based medicine is neither old-hat nor impossible to practice. The argument that everyone already is doing it falls before evidence of striking variations in both the integration of patient values into our clinical behaviour [7] and in the rates with which clinicians provide interventions to their patients [8]. The difficulties that clinicians face in keeping abreast of all the medical advances reported in primary journals are obvious from a comparison of the time required for reading (for general medicine, enough to examine

Introduction

19 articles per day, 365 days per year [9]) with the time available (well under an hour per week by British medical consultants, even on self-reports [10]).

The argument that evidence-based medicine can be conducted only from ivory towers and armchairs is refuted by audits in the front lines of clinical care where at least some inpatient clinical teams in general medicine [11], psychiatry (JR Geddes *et al.*, Royal College of Psychiatrists winter meeting, January 1996), and surgery (P McCulloch, personal communication) have provided evidence-based care to the vast majority of their patients. Such studies show that busy clinicians who devote their scarce reading time to selective, efficient, patient-driven searching, appraisal and incorporation of the best available evidence can practice evidence-based medicine.

Evidence-based medicine is not "cook-book" medicine. Because it requires a bottom-up approach that integrates the best external evidence with individual clinical expertise and patient-choice, it cannot result in slavish, cook-book approaches to individual patient care. External clinical evidence can inform, but can never replace, individual clinical expertise, and it is this expertise that decides whether the external evidence applies to the individual patient at all and, if so, how it should be integrated into a clinical decision. Similarly, any external guideline must be integrated with individual clinical expertise in deciding whether and how it matches the patient's clinical state, predicament, and preferences, and thus whether it should be applied. Clinicians who fear top-down cook-books will find the advocates of evidence-based medicine joining them at the barricades.

Evidence-based medicine is not cost-cutting medicine. Some fear that evidence-based medicine will be hijacked by purchasers and managers to cut the costs of health care. This would not only be a misuse of evidence-based medicine but suggests a fundamental misunderstanding of its financial consequences. Doctors practising evidence-based medicine will identify and apply the most efficacious interventions to maximise the quality and quantity of life for individual patients; this may raise rather than lower the cost of their care.

Evidence-based medicine is not restricted to randomised trials and meta-analyses. It involves tracking down the best external evidence with which to answer our clinical questions. To find out about the accuracy of a diagnostic test, we need to find proper cross-sectional studies of patients clinically suspected of harbouring the relevant disorder, not a randomised trial. For a question about prognosis, we need proper follow-up studies of patients assembled at a uniform, early point in the clinical course of their disease. And sometimes the evidence we need will come from the basic sciences such as genetics or immunology. It is when asking questions about therapy that we should try to avoid the non-experimental approaches, since these routinely lead to false-positive conclusions about efficacy. Because the randomised trial, and especially the systematic review of several randomised trials, is so much more likely to inform us and so much less likely to mislead us, it has become the "gold standard" for judging whether a treatment does more good than harm. However, some questions about therapy do not require randomised trials (successful interventions for otherwise fatal conditions) or cannot wait for the trials to be conducted. And if no randomised trial has been carried out for our patient's predicament, we follow the trail to the next best external evidence and work from there.

Despite its ancient origins, evidence-based medicine remains a relatively young discipline whose positive impacts are just beginning to be validated [12, 13], and it will continue to evolve. This evolution will be enhanced as several undergraduate, post-graduate, and continuing medical education programmes adopt and adapt it to their learners' needs. These programmes, and their evaluation, will provide further information and understanding about what evidence-based medicine is, and what it is not.

References

1 British Medical Association: *Report of the working party on medical education*. London: British Medical Association, 1995.

2 Standing Committee on Postgraduate Medical and Dental Education: *Creating a better learning environment in hospitals: 1 Teaching hospital doctors and dentists to teach*. London: SCOPME, 1994.

3 General Medical Council: *Education Committee Report*. London: General Medical Council, 1994.

4 Grahame-Smith D: Evidence-based medicine: Socratic dissent. *BMJ* 1995; 310: 1126–7.

5 Evidence-based medicine, in its place (editorial). *Lancet* 1995; 346: 785.

6 Correspondence. Evidence-based Medicine. *Lancet* 1995; 346: 1171–2.

7 Weatherall DJ: The inhumanity of medicine. *BMJ* 1994; 308: 1671–2.

8 House of Commons Health Committee. *Priority setting in the NHS: purchasing*. First report sessions 1994–95. London: HMSO, 1995, (HC 134–1.)

9 Davidoff F, Haynes B, Sackett D, Smith R: Evidence-based medicine; a new journal to help doctors identify the information they need. *BMJ* 1995; 310: 1085–6.

10 Sackett DL: Surveys of self-reported reading times of consultants in Oxford, Birmingham, Milton-Keynes, Bristol, Leicester, and Glasgow, 1995. In Rosenberg WMC, Richardson WS, Haynes RB, Sackett DL. *Evidence-based Medicine*. London: Churchill-Livingstone, 1999.

11 Ellis J, Mulligan I, Rowe J, Sackett DL: Inpatient general medicine is evidence based. *Lancet* 1995; 346: 407–10.

12 Bennett RJ, Sackett DL, Haynes RB, Neufeld VR: A controlled trial of teaching critical appraisal of the clinical literature to medical students. *JAMA* 1987; 257: 2451–4.

13 Shin JH, Haynes RB, Johnston ME: Effect of problem-based, self-directed undergraduate education on life-long learning. *Can Med Assoc J* 1993; 148: 969–76.

Critical appraisal of a clinical article about therapy

A 37-year old businessman attends your morning surgery. He complains of four days of profuse diarrhoea with abdominal cramps. This has responded somewhat to loperamide bought from the chemist, but he is still passing loose stools 4–5 times daily, and he is worried about how he will cope with his week, in which he is scheduled to drive several hundred miles to attend meetings with clients. On examination, he is afebrile and abdominal examination is not worrying. You remember an editorial in the *British Medical Journal* suggesting that ciprofloxacin could help with community-acquired diarrhoea. You feel under pressure to do something active for your patient, and write out a prescription. After he has left, you wonder whether this was the best thing to do, and form the clinical question: 'In patients with community-acquired diarrhoea, does empiric treatment with ciprofloxacin reduce the duration of the illness, in comparison to symptomatic treatments alone?'

You manage to find the editorial which had originally recommended the use of ciprofloxacin, but this does not contain the evidence you are looking for. However, the editorial does reference its recommendations to a journal article. The journal is not one to which you have ready access, but on telephoning the local hospital library, you learn that they stock it and they agree to fax a copy to you: *Clinical Infectious Diseases* (1996) **22:** 1019–25. You could also have found this article by searching MEDLINE using the free text terms 'ciprofloxacin' and 'diarrhea'. (But note that if you had used the English spelling (diarrhoea) the article would not have been retrieved. Entering diarr* is a way of overcoming this problem when you know that English and American spellings differ.)

Read the article and decide:
1   Is the evidence from this randomised trial valid?
2   If valid, is this evidence important?
3   If valid and important, can you apply this evidence in caring for your patient?

If you want to read some strategies for answering these sorts of questions, you could have a look at pp 91–6, 133–41 and 166–72 in *Evidence-based Medicine*.

1 We illustrate the importance, strategies and tactics of formulating clinical questions and work with you on the three to four parts of the question.
2 Participants break up into groups of two, discuss patients they cared for in the previous week, and generate questions they think are important concerning their patients' therapy, diagnosis and prognosis.
3 In larger groups, we review and refine the questions, and then keep track of them as possible questions to use in later sessions devoted to searching for the best evidence.

Empirical Treatment of Severe Acute Community-Acquired Gastroenteritis with Ciprofloxacin

Matthew S. Dryden, Richard J. E. Gabb, and Sarah K. Wright

From the Department of Microbiology, Royal Hampshire County Hospital, Winchester, Hampshire, United Kingdom

We conducted a randomized controlled trial to determine whether empirical treatment of severe acute community-acquired gastroenteritis (four fluid stools per day for >3 days) with ciprofloxacin reduces the duration of diarrhea and other symptoms and to determine what effect ciprofloxacin has on the duration of long-term fecal carriage of gastrointestinal pathogens. A total of 173 patients were recruited for the study and received either ciprofloxacin (500 mg b.i.d.) or placebo for 5 days, during which time they recorded the duration of diarrhea and other symptoms (fever, abdominal pain, vomiting, and myalgia). Fecal samples were collected before treatment and regularly after treatment to determine the duration of carriage of gastrointestinal pathogens. Antibiotic susceptibility tests were performed, and the minimum inhibitory concentrations (MICs) of ciprofloxacin were determined. A significant reduction in the duration of diarrhea and other symptoms was observed after treatment, regardless of whether a pathogen was detected ($P = .0001$). Treatment failure occurred in 3 of 81 patients in the ciprofloxacin group and 17 of 81 patients in the placebo group. Significant pathogens were detected in 87% of patients, 85.5% of whom had cleared the pathogen at the end of treatment with ciprofloxacin, as compared with 34% who received placebo. Six weeks after treatment, there was no difference between the two groups in terms of the pathogen carriage rate (12%). Treatment with ciprofloxacin did not prolong carriage. High-level resistance to ciprofloxacin (MIC, >32 mg/L) was detected in three strains (4%) of *Campylobacter* species.

Acute gastroenteritis is becoming an increasingly important public health problem [1]. In the United Kingdom, >150,000 official notifications of food poisoning (undoubtedly much lower than the true figure) were made in the 3-year period 1989–1991, and this figure represented a 69% increase over the previous 3-year period. Severe gastroenteritis accounts for considerable morbidity among otherwise healthy persons. Although it is generally a self-limiting illness, it is the cause of a number of deaths each year (541 deaths between 1989 and 1991), usually among patients with other underlying illnesses. Gastroenteritis has both a social and an economic impact and is responsible for loss of productivity at work. Salmonellosis alone is estimated to cost between \$346 and \$496 million annually in the United Kingdom [2].

Acute gastroenteritis may be caused by viruses, bacteria, or protozoa. Viral gastroenteritis is most common, especially in children, and it is short-lived, usually mild, and requires only

supportive therapy. In the United Kingdom, *Campylobacter* species, followed by *Salmonella* species and *Shigella* species, are the most common causes of acute bacterial gastroenteritis. Antibiotic treatment of acute gastroenteritis has generally been discouraged because the disease is usually self-limiting, and often the patient is recovering by the time the microbiological diagnosis is made. Antibiotics are ineffective for viral infections, and the view has long been that antibiotics do not reduce the duration of symptoms of bacterial gastroenteritis [3] and may indeed prolong gastrointestinal carriage of the pathogen [4, 5].

Ciprofloxacin, a fluoroquinolone, is active against all the recognized bacterial causes of gastroenteritis. It concentrates at high levels within the enteric mucosa, does not greatly affect the normal anaerobic bowel flora [6], and penetrates effectively into macrophages [7]; all of these characteristics make this agent an effective drug for treatment of bacterial gastroenteritis. Ciprofloxacin has been effective in the treatment of enteric fever [8–10], traveler's diarrhea [11, 12], and acute diarrhea in patients admitted to the hospital [13] as well as those presenting to the hospital [14]. This drug has also been used with mixed success to clear gastrointestinal carriage of pathogens [15–18]. Most cases of bacterial gastroenteritis are community acquired, and only a minority of patients require hospitalization. Therefore, we studied the efficacy of ciprofloxacin in the treatment of severe acute community-acquired gastroenteritis.

Methods

Patients over the age of 18 who were not pregnant and presented to their general practitioners with severe acute gastro-

Received 14 September 1995; revised 5 January 1996.

This work was presented in part at a conference on gastrointestinal infection held at the Royal Society of Medicine on 28 June 1995 in London.

Informed consent was obtained from the patients, and the study was approved by the ethics committee of the Royal Hampshire County Hospital, Winchester, United Kingdom.

Grant support: Bayer, Newbury, United Kingdom.

Reprints or correspondence: Dr. Matthew Dryden, Department of Microbiology, Royal Hampshire County Hospital, Winchester, Hants, S022 5DG, United Kingdom.

Clinical Infectious Diseases 1996;22:1019–25
© 1996 by The University of Chicago. All rights reserved.
1058–4838/96/2206–0016$02.00

enteritis were recruited for the study. Severe acute gastroenteritis was defined as diarrhea (more than four fluid stools per day) that had not abated in ≥3 days in an otherwise healthy person with at least one of the following symptoms: abdominal pain, fever, vomiting, myalgia, or headache. The severity of these symptoms and the need for parenteral rehydration were not used as inclusion criteria.

Patients were told that they would receive an active agent or placebo in addition to standard supportive therapy (fluids and no food until the return of appetite, followed by bland foods until the return of normal bowel habits). Antiperistaltic drugs were not recommended, but if they were prescribed by the general practitioner, they could be taken as required.

Patients recorded their own symptoms by completing a questionnaire on the date and time of the onset of illness, the last fluid stool, and the time it took (to the nearest half day) for the stool consistency and stool frequency to return to normal. The presence and duration of vomiting, abdominal pain, fever, myalgia, headache, and general malaise were noted. Many patients did not measure their temperatures; therefore, fever was merely defined as feeling hot, shivery, or sweaty. A record was made of underlying illnesses or medications, history of recent travel outside the United Kingdom, and adverse reactions to the treatment. The questionnaire was returned to the investigators after patients recovered.

Patients were randomized to receive placebo or ciprofloxacin (500 mg b.i.d.). Treatment was blinded, and patients were given a numbered tablet container; the list of numbers and which tablets the patients had received was retained by the hospital pharmacy until the end of the study. Placebo and ciprofloxacin tablets were indistinguishable. Compliance was determined by asking patients if they had completed the course of treatment and by requesting return of the numbered tablet container with the questionnaire. Stool samples were collected on recruitment into the study; additional stool samples were requested 2–3 days after the 5-day course of treatment had been completed and again 6 weeks later. Additional stool samples were collected each week from patients in whom carriage of a pathogen persisted.

Patients infected with pathogens such as *Giardia lamblia* or *Entamoeba histolytica,* for which appropriate alternative therapy was available, were excluded from the trial. Patients in whom no pathogens were detected or who were infected with pathogens such as *Cryptosporidium* species, for which no satisfactory treatment exists, remained in the trial. Treatment failure was recorded for patients who had no decrease in the frequency or severity of diarrhea towards the end of the course of treatment or who continued to have severe abdominal pain. Some of these patients were offered alternative therapy at the discretion of their general practitioners; this therapy included ciprofloxacin for those with infections due to *Salmonella* species and *Shigella* species or erythromycin for those with infections due to *Campylobacter* species. In addition, supportive therapy (including parenteral rehydration in the hospital) was offered

when clinically indicated. Patients who received additional therapy were not included in the analysis of the duration of illness or duration of gastrointestinal carriage of pathogens, but they were included in the comparison of treatment failures.

Stool samples were processed in the microbiology laboratory with use of routine methods. Samples were inoculated on deoxycholate citrate agar (DCA; bioMérieux, Basingstoke, England), on xylose-lysine-deoxycholate agar (XLD; bioMérieux), and in selenite broth and incubated aerobically at 37°C for 18–24 hours; they were also inoculated on campylobacter blood-free selective agar (Oxoid; Basingstoke) and incubated under microaerophilic conditions at 37°C. Microscopic examinations for ova, cysts, and parasites (including a phenol auramine stain for detection of *Cryptosporidium* species) was performed. Significant isolates were identified by means of routine methods. *Campylobacter* isolates were identified to the species level on the basis of their ability to hydrolyze hippurate.

Antibiotic susceptibility was determined by a disk diffusion method [18] with use of amoxicillin (25 μg), trimethoprim (2.5 μg), chloramphenicol (10 μg), cefuroxime (30 μg), gentamicin (10 μg), and ciprofloxacin (5 μg) for species of *Salmonella, Shigella,* and *Aeromonas* and erythromycin (5 μg), nalidixic acid (30 μg), and ciprofloxacin (5 μg) for species of *Campylobacter.* MICs of ciprofloxacin were determined for all isolates by an agar diffusion method (E test; Difco, East Molesey, Surrey, United Kingdom).

Data were recorded in a file (Dbase IV, Borland, CA) by patient number. The data analyzed included age, sex, pathogen isolated, total duration of symptoms, duration of diarrhea after the start of treatment, duration of other symptoms after the start of treatment, presence of the pathogen immediately after discontinuation of treatment, and persistence of the pathogen 6 weeks after discontinuation of treatment. At the end of the study, a separate file containing the treatment coding was combined with the main clinical data file. The duration of diarrhea and other symptoms in the two groups was compared by the Wilcoxon two-sample test. Statistical comparison of treatment failure in the two groups was performed by means of the χ^2 test.

Results

One hundred and seventy-three patients were recruited for the study. Eleven of these patients were excluded for the following reasons: one patient concurrently received other antibiotics, eight failed to comply with the therapeutic protocol, and two had diagnoses other than gastroenteritis (inflammatory bowel disease and giardiasis). Patients were not excluded for failure to provide any of the three stool samples, but those who did not provide the necessary sample were rigourously encouraged to do so.

Eighty-one patients could be evaluated in each arm of the trial. There were no statistical differences between the two groups of patients in terms of age, sex, history of travel, or

Table 1. Characteristics and presenting symptoms of patients with severe acute community-acquired gastroenteritis who received ciprofloxacin or placebo.

Variable	No. of patients with indicated characteristic	
	Ciprofloxacin group ($n = 81$)*	Placebo group ($n = 81$)*
Sex		
Male	38	37
Female	43	44
History of travel outside the United Kingdom	17	23
Symptoms		
Fever	57	51
Vomiting	32	21
Abdominal pain	75	71
Myalgia	46	37

* The mean age of patients in the ciprofloxacin group was 39.8 years (range, 19–73 years), and that of patients in the placebo group was 43.4 years (range, 19–81 years).

Table 2. Pathogens isolated from patients with severe acute community-acquired gastroenteritis.

Pathogen	No. of patients infected with indicated pathogen	
	Ciprofloxacin group ($n = 81$)	Placebo group ($n = 81$)
Aeromonas sobria	0	1
Campylobacter jejuni	30	31
Campylobacter coli	6	7
Campylobacter jejuni and *C. coli*	1	0
Salmonella enteritidis phage type 4	18	18
S. enteritidis (other phage types)	2	1
Salmonella virchow	4	2
Salmonella hadar	0	2
Salmonella ouakam	0	1
Salmonella senftenberg	0	1
Salmonella chester	0	1
Shigella flexneri	3	1
Shigella sonnei	4	3
S. sonnei and *Aeromonas* species	1	0
Salmonella species and *Aeromonas* species	0	1
Vibrio cholerae non-O1	1	0
Cryptosporidium species	1	0
None	10	11

presenting symptoms (table 1), and there was no difference between the groups in terms of the use of antidiarrheal agents. These agents included loperamide (11 patients in the ciprofloxacin group and 16 in the placebo group), kaolin and morphine (3 in the ciprofloxacin group and 1 in the placebo group), and codeine phosphate (5 in the ciprofloxacin group and 4 in the placebo group). The mean ($\pm$SD) duration of diarrhea before commencing treatment was 4.4 $\pm$ 1.7 days for the ciprofloxacin group and 4.2 $\pm$ 1.2 days for the placebo group. Pathogens were detected by microbiological examination of stools for 71 (88%) patients receiving ciprofloxacin and 70 (86%) receiving placebo (table 2). There were no statistical differences between the two groups in terms of the isolation rates for pathogens. *Campylobacter* species were the most commonly detected pathogens (75 patients [46%]) followed by *Salmonella* species, 51 patients [31%]). No pathogens were detected in 21 patients (13%)

For the patients in the ciprofloxacin group, the duration of diarrhea and other symptoms was significantly shorter after treatment ($P < .0001$; table 3). Cumulative recovery is shown in figure 1. Ciprofloxacin treatment reduced the duration of symptoms regardless of whether a pathogen was detected or whether its identity was determined (figure 2). For patients whose symptoms did not resolve, treatment failure was recorded. There were three treatment failures in the ciprofloxacin group, compared with 17 in the placebo group ($P < .001$). One patient in the ciprofloxacin group and four in the placebo group received alternative antimicrobial therapy after treatment failure was recorded. These patients were not included in the analysis of duration of infection and carriage.

At the end of the 5-day course of treatment, follow-up stool samples were obtained from 69 of 71 patients in the ciproflox-

acin group who had pathogens isolated and 67 of 70 in the placebo group who had pathogens isolated. Fifty-nine patients (85.5%) had cleared the pathogen in the ciprofloxacin group, compared with 23 (34%) in the placebo group (table 4). Six weeks after treatment, final follow-up stool samples were obtained from 67 patients in the ciprofloxacin group and 65 in the placebo group. The fecal carriage rate was the same in both groups: 8 (11.9%) of patients in the ciprofloxacin group were carriers, and 8 (12.3%) of those in the placebo group were

Table 3. Duration of symptoms in patients with severe acute community-acquired gastroenteritis who received ciprofloxacin or placebo.

Symptom	Mean (range) duration of symptoms in days		
	Ciprofloxacin group	Placebo group	P value
Diarrhea (after treatment)	2.2 (1.7–2.7)	4.6 (3.6–5.2)	<.0001
Other symptoms*	1.9 (1.5–2.3)	4.3 (3.5–5.1)	<.0001
Total no. of days diarrhea and/or other symptoms were present	7 (6.2–7.8)	8.3 (6.5–10.1)	.082

* Fever, vomiting, and abdominal pain.

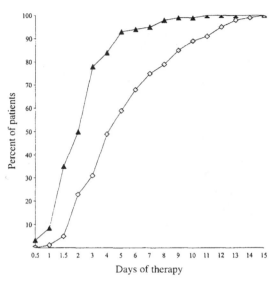

Figure 1. Cumulative recovery from diarrhea among patients with severe acute gastroenteritis who received ciprofloxacin (▲) or placebo (◇).

carriers. These patients were followed up by means of weekly examinations of stool samples. Carriage persisted for a mean of 10.3 weeks (range, 7–20 weeks) in the ciprofloxacin group and 11.5 weeks (range, 9–18 weeks) in the placebo group. There was no significant difference in the patterns of carriage rates among the subsets of patients infected with specific organisms (table 4).

In no case was a pathogen detected after discontinuation of therapy in patients who had had negative fecal microbiology on admission to the trial. For one patient who received ciprofloxacin, the pathogen was not detected at the end of treatment but was present 6 weeks later. This patient, who was subsequently found to have hairy-cell leukemia, developed septicemia and splenic abscess caused by *Salmonella enteritidis* 2 months after leukemia was diagnosed.

All but three isolates were susceptible to ciprofloxacin; these three isolates were *Campylobacter* species for which the MICs of ciprofloxacin were >32 mg/L. Only one of these infections was acquired abroad (Majorca). Two of the patients received placebo and recovered without further treatment; the third received ciprofloxacin, and although the diarrhea resolved after 4 days, the patient continued to have severe abdominal pain, which was considered treatment failure. This patient was given erythromycin. The organism continued to be isolated from the patient's stool after ciprofloxacin therapy but was absent 6 weeks after treatment with erythromycin.

No demonstrable resistance developed during treatment. A susceptible strain of *Campylobacter jejuni* (MIC of ciprofloxa-

cin, 0.125 mg/L) was detected in a pretreatment stool sample from one patient who was found to have a resistant *Campylobacter* strain (MIC of ciprofloxacin, >32 mg/L) at the end of treatment. However, the isolate recovered after treatment was identified as *Campylobacter coli*. Presumably, both strains were present before treatment, but only the susceptible one was detected.

The MICs of ciprofloxacin for species of *Salmonella* and *Shigella* were low (range, 0.006–0.094 mg/L) (figure 3). Only 9 (37.5%) of 24 isolates acquired abroad vs. 36 (92.3%) of 39 isolates acquired in the United Kingdom were fully susceptible to all the antibiotics tested. Twenty-eight percent of *Salmonella* and *Shigella* isolates were resistant to amoxicillin, 19% were resistant to trimethoprim, and 6.3% were resistant to chloramphenicol. Resistance to cefuroxime or gentamicin was not demonstrated. The MICs of ciprofloxacin for isolates of *Campylobacter* species were higher (range, 0.016–>32 mg/L) (figure 3). Only 3 (4.2%) of 72 isolates were resistant to nalidixic acid and ciprofloxacin. Resistance to erythromycin was not demonstrated.

Ciprofloxacin therapy was well tolerated, with few reported adverse effects. Eight patients reported adverse effects; only two of these adverse effects could be attributed to ciprofloxacin and included an unpleasant taste and vaginal thrush. Other adverse effects reported in the ciprofloxacin group included "short temper," "muscle jumping," "swollen, painful second finger," and "felt sick," and those reported in the placebo group included "felt sick" and, surprisingly, "constipation."

Discussion

This study demonstrated that a 5-day course of therapy with oral ciprofloxacin reduces the duration of diarrhea and other symptoms in patients with severe acute community-acquired gastroenteritis. A reduction in the duration of symptoms was observed regardless of whether a pathogen was detected. Most gastroenteritis is short-lived, self-limiting, and clinically mild. Such cases clearly do not require antibiotic therapy. Gastroenteritis is generally perceived as a self-limiting illness, and patients tend not to consult a physician unless the illness persists.

It is likely that the patients in this trial represented the more-severe end of the spectrum of community-acquired gastroenteritis. On average, they had been unwell for just over 4 days before seeking the help of a physician, and therefore their illnesses were unlikely to have been of viral etiology. The relatively late presentation of these patients makes a bacterial etiology more likely and explains the high rate (87%) of detection of gastrointestinal pathogens in the trial. Such patients are the ones who will benefit from empirical therapy.

Bacterial gastroenteritis in healthy persons is uncomfortable and disrupts their life. The average duration of illness in untreated patients in this study was ~1 week; therefore, if treatment reduces symptoms by a few days, it is worthwhile, particularly when it is safe and well tolerated.

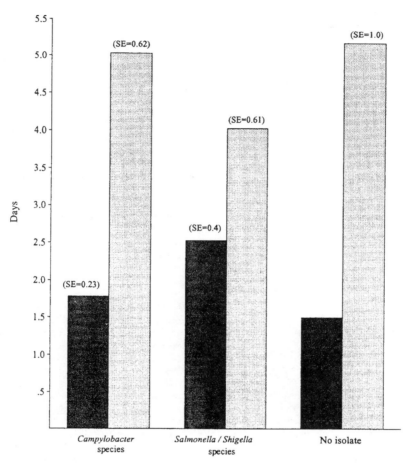

Figure 2. Mean duration of diarrhea in days after starting treatment with ciprofloxacin (■) or placebo (☐).

Gastroenteritis results in considerable morbidity, some mortality, and extensive costs in terms of loss of wages and reduced productivity [2, 16]; thus, an effective empirical treatment would be helpful. The general practitioner rarely has the luxury of knowing the etiologic agent when faced with a sick patient. Antibiotic treatment of gastroenteritis was previously discouraged because of its poor efficacy in patients with this condition [3]; however, with the advent of the quinolones, this has changed.

Considerable experience with the quinolones in the treatment of gastrointestinal infection has been amassed worldwide, and most investigators have found the quinolones to be effective. Many of the studies have examined patients who have been admitted to the hospital [13] or who are in the hospital for treatment of specific infections such as shigellosis [20]. These studies have shown that therapy with the quinolones reduces the duration of symptoms. Empirical treatment of community-acquired diarrhea with ciprofloxacin in urban American adults showed that a 5-day course was more effective in reducing the duration of diarrhea than was therapy with co-trimoxazole [14]. In a multinational study conducted in Latin America and Italy, norfloxacin was found to be more effective than co-trimoxazole [21], and the cure rate was higher when the patient's stool sample contained leukocytes. Ciprofloxacin has been used successfully to treat typhoid [8, 10] and traveler's diarrhea [11, 12].

If ciprofloxacin is to be administered empirically for gastroenteritis, who should receive it? Patients with proven bacterial gastroenteritis have a more-severe illness than do those from whom no pathogens are recovered [14]. Ciprofloxacin therapy should be reserved for adults who have unremitting diarrhea (more than four fluid stools per day) for >3 days and who have

Table 4. Eradication of pathogens among patients with severe acute gastroenteritis who received ciprofloxacin or placebo.

Time of detection of pathogen	No. of patients with pathogen detected at indicated time		P value
	Ciprofloxacin group (n = 81)	Placebo group (n = 81)	
Pathogens detected at start of treatment			
All cases	71	70	
Salmonella/Shigella species	31	30	
Campylobacter species	36	38	
Pathogen still present after treatment			
All cases	10*	44*	<.0001
Salmonella/Shigella species	5	23	
Campylobacter species	4	21	
Pathogen still present 6 weeks after treatment			
All cases	8†	8†	.94
Salmonella/Shigella species	6	5	
Campylobacter species	2	3	

* Follow-up stool samples were obtained from 69 patients in the ciprofloxacin group and 67 in the placebo group.
† Final follow-up stool samples were obtained from 67 patients in the ciprofloxacin group and 65 in the placebo group.

had at least one of the following symptoms: fever (temperature, >38°C), vomiting, abdominal pain, or myalgia. The drug should be used as a adjunct to appropriate supportive therapy, particularly fluid replacement. A stool sample should always be collected before the initiation of treatment so that the diagnosis can be confirmed, epidemiological information can be provided, and other treatable infections such as giardiasis or amebiasis can be excluded.

In the present study, ciprofloxacin was effective even in those patients from whom a pathogen was not recovered. The negative microbiological results could be explained in one of several ways: the laboratory failed to detect the pathogen, the patient was infected by a susceptible pathogen not routinely sought (e.g., a pathogenic strain of *Escherichia coli* or *Yersinia* species), or the patient was infected by a susceptible but as yet unrecognized pathogen.

The rate of pathogen eradication immediately after treatment was significantly higher in the ciprofloxacin group. The present study did not address the problem of microbiological relapse in the short term, which is of little significance to the patient providing symptoms have abated. Six weeks after treatment, there was no difference between the two groups in terms of the carriage rates. Follow-up of the persistent carriers did not demonstrate any difference between the groups in duration of carriage; thus, ciprofloxacin did not prolong pathogen carriage,

as is widely believed to be the case following treatment with other antibiotics [6]. Ciprofloxacin therapy has been somewhat successful in eradicating carriage in symptomatic and asymptomatic excreters in a number of nosocomial outbreaks [6]. Indeed, during an outbreak in our own hospital, ciprofloxacin therapy eliminated carriage of *S. enteritidis* in asymptomatic catering staff; no relapse was observed up to 6 weeks after therapy [18].

It is therefore surprising that two studies have reported unacceptable rates of microbiological relapse. In the first study, ciprofloxacin was used to eliminate fecal carriage of *Salmonella java* in health care workers [16]. Treatment was started 9 days after the onset of illness, by which time most patients had no symptoms. The pathogen was rapidly cleared after therapy was begun. However, 2–3 weeks after treatment was discontinued, bacteriologic relapse was documented for four of seven patients.

Possible explanations for this relapse may be the late initiation of treatment or the pathogenicity of the *Salmonella* strain. In an open study, norfloxacin therapy cleared *Salmonella typhimurium* in 21 of 23 patients on the last day of a 7-day course; however, 10 of the patients had a subsequent bacteriologic relapse [17]. In neither of these studies did the quinolone unequivocally prolong carriage, nor was relapse associated with resistance of the pathogen. Since the pathogen was eventually eradicated naturally, the significance of its persistence in terms of public health is negligible, providing the patient practices good personal hygiene.

Ciprofloxacin has been shown in vitro to have a high degree of activity against a wide range of gastrointestinal pathogens from a variety of geographic locations [22]. The majority of the pathogens in the present study were susceptible to ciprofloxacin. No resistance to ciprofloxacin was detected among species of *Salmonella* and *Shigella*. Resistance to other antibiotics was more common in these organisms if the infection had been acquired outside the United Kingdom; resistance to amoxicillin and trimethoprim was most common. However, two of the three ciprofloxacin-resistant *Campylobacter* isolates

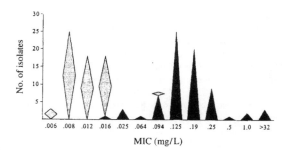

Figure 3. MIC (mg/L) of ciprofloxacin for isolates of *Salmonella* and/or *Shigella* (◆) and *Campylobacter* (▲) from patients with severe acute gastroenteritis.

were acquired in the United Kingdom, and both were highly resistant to the drug; the MICs of ciprofloxacin for these organisms were >32 mg/L. It has been shown that such high-level resistance to quinolones in other organisms emerges after prolonged exposure to the agent [23]. In the case of *Campylobacter* species, selective pressure is likely to have been due to antibiotic use in the agricultural setting [24], although the development of high-level resistance has occurred during treatment of gastroenteritis [25]. The use of quinolones in animal husbandry is of concern. There is no evidence that these drugs reduce the pathogen load in raw meat products, and resistance to quinolones could emerge in other organisms that enter the food chain, limiting the usefulness of these agents in the treatment of human infections.

The question remains as to whether the reduction (~2 days) in duration of symptoms warrants the recommendation that otherwise healthy patients with severe gastroenteritis be treated empirically with ciprofloxacin. Both medically and socioeconomically, such a reduction in the duration of symptoms is likely to be worthwhile. Further work is required to establish the true economic impact. It is also possible that a shorter course of ciprofloxacin therapy would be as effective, as has been demonstrated among patients with traveler's diarrhea [12].

Acknowledgment

The authors are grateful to the general practitioners in the Winchester, Andover, and Eastleigh areas of Hampshire, United Kingdom, for their help in recruiting patients and for their support throughout the study.

References

1. Sockett PN, Cowden JM, Le Baigue S, Ross D, Adak GK, Evans H. Foodborne disease surveillance in England and Wales: 1989–1991. Commun Dis Rep CDR Rev 1993;3:R159–73.
2. Sockett PN, Roberts JA. The social and economic impact of salmonellosis. A report of a national survey in England and Wales of laboratory-confirmed salmonella infections. Epidemiol Infect 1991;107:335–47.
3. Levine MM. Antimicrobial therapy for infectious diarrhea. Rev Infect Dis 1986;8(suppl 2):S207–16.
4. Dixon JMS. Effect of antibiotic treatment on duration of excretion of *Salmonella typhimurium* by children. Br Med J 1965;2:1343–5.
5. Aserkoff B, Bennett JV. Effect of antibiotic therapy in acute salmonellosis on the fecal excretion of salmonellae. N Engl J Med 1969;281:636–40.
6. Nathwani D, Wood MJ. Ciprofloxacin and salmonella carriage [editorial]. J Hosp Infect 1992;22:181–4.
7. Easmon CS, Crane JP, Blowers A. Effect of ciprofloxacin on intracellular organisms: in-vitro and in-vivo studies. J Antimicrob Chemother 1986; 18 (suppl D):43–8.
8. Eykyn SJ, Williams H. Treatment of multiresistant *Salmonella typhi* with oral ciprofloxacin [letter]. Lancet 1987;2:1407–8.
9. Stanley PJ, Flegg PJ, Madal BK, Geddes AM. Open study of ciprofloxacin in enteric fever. J Antimicrob Chemother 1989;23:789–91.
10. Pithie AD, Wood MJ. Treatment of typhoid fever and infectious diarrhoea with ciprofloxacin. J Antimicrob Chemother 1990;26(suppl F):47–53.
11. Ericsson CD, Johnson PC, Dupont HL, Morgan DR, Bitsura JA, Javier de la Cabada FJ. Ciprofloxacin or trimethoprim-sulfamethoxazole as initial therapy for travelers' diarrhea: a placebo-controlled, randomized trial. Ann Intern Med 1987;106:216–20.
12. Salam I, Katelaris P, Leigh-Smith S, Farthing MJ. Randomised trial of single-dose ciprofloxacin for travellers' diarrhoea. Lancet 1994;344: 1537–9.
13. Pichler HE, Diridl G, Stickler K, Wolf D. Clinical efficacy of ciprofloxacin compared with placebo in bacterial diarrhea. Am J Med 1987;82(A4): 329–32.
14. Goodman LJ, Trenholme GM, Kaplan RL, et al. Empiric antimicrobial therapy of domestically acquired acute diarrhea in urban adults. Arch Intern Med 1990;150:541–6.
15. Ulutan F. Effect of quinolones on the duration of salmonella carriage after acute salmonellosis [letter]. Scand J Infect Dis 1991;23:513–4.
16. Neill MA, Opal SM, Heelan J, et al. Failure of ciprofloxacin to eradicate convalescent fecal excretion after acute salmonellosis: experience during an outbreak in health care workers. Ann Intern Med 1991;114: 195–9.
17. Carlstedt G, Dahl P, Niklasson PM, Gullberg K, Banck G, Kahlmeter G. Norfloxacin treatment of salmonellosis does not shorten the carrier stage. Scand J Infect Dis 1990;22:553–6.
18. Dryden MS, Keyworth N, Gabb R, Stein K. Asymptomatic foodhandlers as the source of nosocomial salmonellosis. J Hosp Infect 1994;28:195–208.
19. Phillips I. A guide to sensitivity testing. British Society of Antimicrobial Chemotherapy. London: Academic Press, 1991.
20. Bennish ML, Salam MA, Haider R, Barza M. Therapy for shigellosis. II. Randomized, double-blind comparison of ciprofloxacin and ampicillin. J Infect Dis 1990;162:711–6.
21. DuPont HL, Corrado ML, Sabbaj J. Use of norfloxacin in the treatment of acute diarrheal disease. Am J Med 1987;82(6B):79–83.
22. DuPont HL, Ericsson CD, Robinson A, Johnson PC. Current problems in antimicrobial therapy for bacterial enteric infection. Am J Med 1987; 82(A4):324–8.
23. Dryden MS, Talsania H, McCann M, Cookson BD, Phillips I. The epidemiology of ciprofloxacin resistance in coagulase-negative staphylococci in CAPD patients. Epidemiol Infect 1992;109:97–112.
24. Endtz HP, Moutoun RP, van der Reyden T, Ruijs GJ, Biever M, van Klingeren B. Fluoroquinolone resistance in *Campylobacter* spp. isolated from human stools and poultry products [letter]. Lancet 1990;335:787.
25. Segreti J, Gootz TD, Goodman LJ, et al. High-level quinolone resistance in clinical isolates of *Campylobacter jejuni*. J Infect Dis 1992;165:667–70.

Citation:

Are the results of this single preventive or therapeutic trial valid?

Was the assignment of patients to treatments
randomised?
Was the randomisation list concealed?

Were all patients who entered the trial accounted
for at its conclusion?
Were they analysed in the groups to which they
were randomised?

Were patients and clinicians kept 'blind' to which
treatment was being received?

Aside from the experimental treatment, were the
groups treated equally?

Were the groups similar at the start of the trial?

Are the valid results of this randomised trial important?

SAMPLE CALCULATIONS (*see* pp134–40 of *Evidence-based Medicine*). Appropriate if outcomes are
dichotomous – either an outcome occurred or it did not.

Occurrence of diabetic neuropathy		Relative risk reduction (RRR)	Absolute risk reduction (ARR)	Number needed to treat (NNT)
Usual insulin control event rate (CER)	Intensive insulin experimental event rate (EER)	$\dfrac{CER - EER}{CER}$	CER – EER	1/ARR
9.6%	2.8%	$\dfrac{9.6\% - 2.8\%}{9.6\%}$ = 71%	9.6% – 2.8% = 6.8%	1/6.8% = 15 pts

95% confidence interval (CI) on an NNT = 1 / (limits on the CI of its ARR) =

$$+/-1.96\sqrt{\frac{CER \times (1-CER)}{\#\ of\ control\ pts} + \frac{EER \times (1-EER)}{\#\ of\ exper.\ pts}} = +/-1.96\sqrt{\frac{0.096 \times 0.904}{730} + \frac{0.028 \times 0.972}{711}} = +/-2.4\%$$

Are the valid results of this randomised trial important?

YOUR CALCULATIONS Hint: the main results in this paper are recorded as continuous variables (e.g. duration of symptoms), and therefore cannot be expressed in the form in this table. However, in the text the authors do give their results as treatment 'successes' and 'failures' at the end of the treatment period. Those figures could be entered in this table.

		Relative risk reduction (RRR)	Absolute risk reduction (ARR)	Number needed to treat (NNT)
CER	EER	$\dfrac{\text{CER} - \text{EER}}{\text{CER}}$	CER − EER	1/ARR

Can you apply this valid, important evidence about a treatment in caring for your patient?

Do these results apply to your patient?

Is your patient so different from those in the trial that its results can't help you?

How great would the potential benefit of therapy actually be for your individual patient?

Method I: **f**

Risk of the outcome in your patient, relative to patients in the trial.
Expressed as a decimal: _____
NNT/f = _____/_____ =
_____
(NNT for patients like yours)

Method II: **1 / (PEER x RRR)**

Your patient's expected event rate if they received the control treatment: PEER:
1 / (PEER x RRR) = 1/_____ = _____
(NNT for patients like yours)

Are your patient's values and preferences satisfied by the regimen and its consequences?

Do your patient and you have a clear assessment of their values and preferences?

Are they met by this regimen and its consequences?

Additional notes

Citation: Dryden M *et al.* (1996) Empirical treatment of severe acute community-acquired gastroenteritis with ciprofloxacin. *Clinical Infectious Diseases.* 22: 1019–25.

Are the results of this single preventive or therapeutic trial valid?

Was the assignment of patients to treatments randomised?	**Yes.**
Was the randomisation list concealed?	**Yes, held by the hospital pharmacy.**
Were all patients who entered the trial accounted for at its conclusion? Were they analysed in the groups to which they were randomised?	**All were described. However, 11 of 173 patients were excluded from the analysis because they received other antibiotics, failed to comply with therapy or had alternative diagnoses. The analysis was therefore not by intention to treat, and is a possible source of bias.**
Were patients and clinicians kept 'blind' to which treatment was being received?	**Yes.**
Aside from the experimental treatment, were the groups treated equally?	**Yes, each could receive supportive treatments according to the clinical judgement of their doctors.**
Were the groups similar at the start of the trial?	**Yes.**

Are the valid results of this randomised trial important?

SAMPLE CALCULATIONS (see pp134–40 of *Evidence-based Medicine*)

Occurrence of diabetic neuropathy		Relative risk reduction (RRR)	Absolute risk reduction (ARR)	Number needed to treat (NNT)
CER	EER	$\dfrac{\text{CER} - \text{EER}}{\text{CER}}$	CER − EER	1/ARR
9.6%	2.8%	$\dfrac{9.6\% - 2.8\%}{9.6\%}$ $= 71\%$	9.6% − 2.8% = 6.8%	1/6.8% = 15 pts

95% confidence interval (CI) on an NNT = 1 / (limits on the CI of its ARR) =

$$+/-1.96\sqrt{\frac{\text{CER} \times (1-\text{CER})}{\#\text{ of control pts}} + \frac{\text{EER} \times (1-\text{EER})}{\#\text{ of exper. pts}}} = +/-1.96\sqrt{\frac{0.096 \times 0.904}{730} + \frac{0.028 \times 0.972}{711}} = +/-2.4\%$$

YOUR CALCULATIONS

In the text, the authors state that 4/81 (5%) in the ciprofloxacin group and 17/81 (21%) in the placebo group were treatment failures.

		Relative risk reduction (RRR)	Absolute risk reduction (ARR)	Number needed to treat (NNT)
CER	EER	$\dfrac{\text{CER} - \text{EER}}{\text{CER}}$	CER − EER	1/ARR
0.21	0.05	0.76	0.16 (0.06–0.26)	6 (4–16)

95% CI on the ARR = +/–10%

Can you apply this valid, important evidence about a treatment in caring for your patient?

Do these results apply to your patient?

Is your patient so different from those in the trial that its results can't help you?	**No. Our patient is very similar to the patients recruited into the trial.**
How great would the potential benefit of therapy actually be for your individual patient?	**The treatment will probably reduce the duration of his diarrhoea by a couple of days.**
Are your patient's values and preferences satisfied by the regimen and its consequences?	
Do your patient and you have a clear assessment of their values and preferences?	**You will have to weigh the benefits shown in this study with other factors, including concern about development of antibiotic resistant bacteria. The value attached to a reduction in symptoms of this magnitude needs to be addressed with this patient.**
Are they met by this regimen and its consequences?	**Needs to be addressed with this individual.**

Additional notes

It would be helpful to know the frequency of ciprofloxacin resistance in countries or communities where the drug is widely prescribed.

Clinical Bottom Line

In patients who have had diarrhoea for more than three days, ciprofloxacin reduces the duration of diarrhoea by about two days. The number needed to treat to prevent continuing symptoms after five days of diarrhoea is 6 (95% CI 4–16).

Citation

Dryden MS, Gabb RJE, Wright SK (1996) Empirical treatment of severe acute community-acquired gastroenteritis with ciprofloxacin. *Clin Infect Dis.* **22**: 1019–25.

Clinical Question

In patients with community-acquired diarrhoea, does empiric treatment with ciprofloxacin reduce the duration of the illness, in comparison to symptomatic treatments alone?

Search Terms

'ciprofloxacin' and 'diarr*' in MEDLINE

The Study

1 Otherwise healthy patients >18 yrs old presenting to GPs in UK with severe acute gastroenteritis (more than four fluid stools/day for three or more days, plus at least one of abdominal pain, fever, vomiting, myalgia or headache.
2 Control group (n = 81): standard supportive therapy (fluids, bland diet, antiperistaltic drugs) and placebo tablets.
3 Experimental group (n = 81): as for control group, plus ciprofloxacin 500 mg twice daily for five days.

The Evidence

The duration of diarrhoea after treatment was begun was 2.4 days less in the ciprofloxacin group than in the control group. This finding was statistically significant, but confidence intervals (or the data to calculate them) were not given.

The authors also present their results as the dichotomous outcome of treatment failure or success at the end of the treatment period. 4/81 (5%) in the ciprofloxacin group and 17/81 (21%) of the placebo group were treatment failures.

CER	EER	Relative risk reduction (RRR)	Absolute risk reduction (ARR)	Number needed to treat (NNT)
CER	EER	$\dfrac{\text{CER} - \text{EER}}{\text{CER}}$	CER – EER	1/ARR
0.21	0.05	0.76	0.16 (0.06–0.26)	6 (4–16)

Comments

1 Analysis was not by intention to treat. Eleven patients were excluded after randomisation and this is a potential bias. *Does it mention which group these were from so that we could do a worst case analysis?*

2 There was no difference in the rate of faecal carriage of organisms after treatment between the experimental and the control group.

3 Side-effects occurred at a similar rate in the two groups.

4 Similar reduction in symptoms with ciprofloxacin was found whether or not a pathogen was subsequently grown from the stool.

5 This study does not address the long-term effects on development of bacteria resistant to ciprofloxacin from its wider use in treating diarrhoea.

Your turn: case-presentations

- Take one of your patients who presented an important problem in therapy, diagnosis, prognosis or harm.

- Formulate that problem into a three-part question (the patient, the manoeuvre and the outcome), based on what you learn from Session 1.

- Do a search for the best evidence based on what you learn from Sessions 3–5 (lots of help available from us or the library team).

- Critically appraise that evidence for its validity, importance, and usefulness.

- Integrate that appraisal with clinical expertise and summarise it (in a one-pager if you wish).

- Present it to the rest of us at one of the final sessions. (Certificates will be given to presenters.)

PART

A Critical appraisal of a clinical article about therapy

A 44-year old woman attends the surgery following the sudden death of her brother aged 47 from a myocardial infarction. You later learn that, although a non-smoker, he was being treated for hypertension and had received dietary advice for a raised cholesterol in the past. She has had no serious illness in the past. She does not smoke, and is not known to have diabetes. She feels that she is overweight and has tried for several years to follow a low-fat diet. Her mother and father, both in their 70s are alive but are being treated for angina. On examination, you find her body mass index is 28 kg/m^2, blood pressure 125/84. Examination of her heart is normal. Review of her records shows that a cholesterol of 6.2 mmol/L was recorded two years ago. You repeat this, and the result is 6.4 mmol/L. HDL cholesterol is 1.0 mmol/L. Her main concern is to know what can be done to reduce her risk of having a heart attack. You identify a raised cholesterol as her main modifiable risk factor.

Together you form the clinical question: 'In a 44-year old woman without a history of cardiovascular disease, does lowering cholesterol with drug treatment lead to a reduction in the risk of myocardial infarction?'

You search *Best Evidence*, using the terms 'cholesterol' and 'myocardial infarction', restricting the search to studies of therapy, and retrieve a relevant article: *NEJM* (1995) **333**(20): 1301–7.

Read the article and decide:
1   Is the evidence from this randomised trial valid?
2   If valid, is this evidence important?
3   If valid and important, can you apply this evidence in caring for your patient?

If you want to read some strategies for answering these sorts of questions, you could have a look at pp 91–6, 133–41 and 166–72 in *Evidence-based Medicine*.

PART

B Asking answerable clinical questions

1   We illustrate the importance, strategies and tactics of formulating clinical questions and work with you on the three to four parts of the question.
2   Participants break up into groups of two, discuss patients they cared for in the previous week, and generate questions they think are important concerning their patients' therapy, diagnosis and prognosis.
3   In larger groups, we review and refine the questions, and then keep track of them as possible questions to use in later sessions devoted to searching for the best evidence.

The New England
Journal of Medicine

©Copyright, 1995, by the Massachusetts Medical Society

Volume 333   NOVEMBER 16, 1995   Number 20

PREVENTION OF CORONARY HEART DISEASE WITH PRAVASTATIN IN MEN WITH HYPERCHOLESTEROLEMIA

James Shepherd, M.D., Stuart M. Cobbe, M.D., Ian Ford, Ph.D., Christopher G. Isles, M.D., A. Ross Lorimer, M.D., Peter W. Macfarlane, Ph.D., James H. McKillop, M.D., and Christopher J. Packard, D.Sc., for the West of Scotland Coronary Prevention Study Group*

Abstract *Background.* Lowering the blood cholesterol level may reduce the risk of coronary heart disease. This double-blind study was designed to determine whether the administration of pravastatin to men with hypercholesterolemia and no history of myocardial infarction reduced the combined incidence of nonfatal myocardial infarction and death from coronary heart disease.

Methods. We randomly assigned 6595 men, 45 to 64 years of age, with a mean (±SD) plasma cholesterol level of 272±23 mg per deciliter (7.0±0.6 mmol per liter) to receive pravastatin (40 mg each evening) or placebo. The average follow-up period was 4.9 years. Medical records, electrocardiographic recordings, and the national death registry were used to determine the clinical end points.

Results. Pravastatin lowered plasma cholesterol levels by 20 percent and low-density lipoprotein cholesterol levels by 26 percent, whereas there was no change with placebo. There were 248 definite coronary events (specified as nonfatal myocardial infarction or death from coro-

nary heart disease) in the placebo group, and 174 in the pravastatin group (relative reduction in risk with pravastatin, 31 percent; 95 percent confidence interval, 17 to 43 percent; $P<0.001$). There were similar reductions in the risk of definite nonfatal myocardial infarctions (31 percent reduction, $P<0.001$), death from coronary heart disease (definite cases alone: 28 percent reduction, $P=0.13$; definite plus suspected cases: 33 percent reduction, $P=0.042$), and death from all cardiovascular causes (32 percent reduction, $P=0.033$). There was no excess of deaths from noncardiovascular causes in the pravastatin group. We observed a 22 percent reduction in the risk of death from any cause in the pravastatin group (95 percent confidence interval, 0 to 40 percent; $P=0.051$).

Conclusions. Treatment with pravastatin significantly reduced the incidence of myocardial infarction and death from cardiovascular causes without adversely affecting the risk of death from noncardiovascular causes in men with moderate hypercholesterolemia and no history of myocardial infarction. (N Engl J Med 1995;333:1301-7.)

EARLIER trials of lipid-lowering drugs in the primary prevention of coronary heart disease have demonstrated that lowering cholesterol levels in middle-aged men with hypercholesterolemia reduces the incidence of myocardial infarction.[1-4] However, these studies, because of their design and low rates of observed events, were unable to show a clear effect of therapy on the risk of death from coronary heart disease or death from any cause. A meta-analysis of the trials provided support for the likelihood that therapy lowered the risk of death from coronary heart disease, but it also aroused concern that the risk of death from noncardiovascular causes might be increased by treat-

ment.[5,6] Whether this latter association was due to chance, to the reduction in cholesterol itself, or to an adverse effect of the drugs is not clear.

Recently, a new class of lipid-lowering drug, the 3-hydroxy-3-methylglutaryl–coenzyme A reductase inhibitors, has been introduced into clinical practice. These drugs block endogenous synthesis of cholesterol and reduce the levels of low-density lipoprotein (LDL) cholesterol. They slow the progression of coronary disease and reduce the incidence of death from coronary causes and death from any cause in men with manifest coronary heart disease.[9-15] The present study was designed to evaluate the effectiveness of a reductase inhibitor, pravastatin (Pravachol), in preventing coronary events in men with moderate hypercholesterolemia and no history of myocardial infarction.

METHODS

Design

The objective was to enroll approximately 6000 middle-aged men, randomly assigned in a double-blind fashion to receive either pravastatin (40 mg each evening) or placebo and to record their clinical progress over a period of five years. The details of the study design,

From the Departments of Pathological Biochemistry (J.S., C.J.P.), Medical Cardiology (S.M.C., A.R.L., P.W.M.), and Medicine (J.H.M.), University of Glasgow and Royal Infirmary, Glasgow; Robertson Centre for Biostatistics, University of Glasgow, Glasgow (I.F.); and the Department of Medicine, Dumfries and Galloway District General Hospital, Dumfries (C.G.I.) — all in Scotland. Address reprint requests to Dr. Ford at the Robertson Centre for Biostatistics, Boyd Orr Bldg., University of Glasgow, Glasgow G12 8QQ, Scotland.

Supported by a research grant from the Bristol-Myers Squibb Pharmaceutical Research Institute, Princeton, N.J.

*The members of the West of Scotland Coronary Prevention Study Group are listed in the Appendix.

Session 1 – Therapy & asking answerable clinical questions

including the definitions of the end points, have been described previously.[16] Briefly, the primary end point of the study was the occurrence of nonfatal myocardial infarction or death from coronary heart disease as a first event; these two categories were combined. Other principal end points were the occurrence of death from coronary heart disease and nonfatal myocardial infarction. In all categories, the events were classified as either definite or suspected. In addition to the main end points, the effect of treatment on death from cardiovascular causes, death from any cause, and the frequency of coronary revascularization procedures was analyzed.

All subjects provided written informed consent. The study was approved by the ethics committees of the University of Glasgow and all participating health boards.

Recruitment and Follow-up

Coronary screening clinics were established in primary medical care facilities throughout the West of Scotland district. Approximately 160,000 men ranging in age from 45 to 64 years were invited to attend the clinics to assess their coronary risk factors. A total of 81,161 appeared for the first visit, and those whose nonfasting plasma cholesterol level was at least 252 mg per deciliter (6.5 mmol per liter) but who had no history of myocardial infarction were given lipid-lowering dietary advice[17] and asked to return four weeks later. A total of 20,914 men returned for the second visit, at which time a lipoprotein profile was obtained that measured plasma cholesterol, the cholesterol content of LDL and high-density lipoprotein (HDL), and plasma triglycerides while the subjects were fasting. If on this occasion the LDL cholesterol level was at least 155 mg per deciliter (4.0 mmol per liter) and the subject had no exclusion criteria,[16] he was advised to stay on the lipid-lowering diet for a further four weeks and then to return for a third visit (13,654 attended), at which time a second lipoprotein profile and a 12-lead electrocardiogram (ECG) were obtained. On the fourth visit the patients underwent randomization if they met the following criteria: fasting LDL cholesterol level of at least 155 mg per deciliter during the second and third visits, with at least one value of 174 mg per deciliter or above (4.5 mmol per liter) and one value of 232 mg per deciliter or below (6.0 mmol per liter); no serious ECG abnormalities according to Minnesota code[18] 1 (pathologic Q waves), 4-1, 5-1, or 7-1-1 or arrhythmia such as atrial fibrillation; and no history of myocardial infarction or other serious illness, although men with stable angina who had not been hospitalized within the previous 12 months were eligible. Further details of the inclusion and exclusion criteria were described previously.[16]

The subjects were seen at three-month intervals, and dietary advice was reinforced on each occasion. A fasting lipoprotein profile was obtained every six months, and an ECG was recorded annually or as required clinically. The subjects received a full medical examination by a physician each year.

Laboratory Analyses

The cholesterol measurement during the first visit was performed on a Reflotron bench-top analyzer (Boehringer–Mannheim, Lewes, Kent, United Kingdom). All subsequent laboratory analyses, including biochemical, hematologic, and lipoprotein profiles, were conducted at the central laboratory at the Glasgow Royal Infirmary. Lipoprotein profiles were determined according to the Lipid Research Clinics protocol[19] with enzymatic cholesterol and triglyceride assays. The laboratory was certified through the Lipid Standardization Program of the Centers for Disease Control and Prevention in Atlanta. Abnormalities in the results of blood tests were identified with the use of published reference ranges.[16]

Siemens Sicard 440 electrocardiographs were used to record the 12-lead ECGs, and the data were transmitted by telephone to the ECG core laboratory at the Glasgow Royal Infirmary for storage on a central Mingocare data base (Siemens Elema, Stockholm, Sweden) and subsequent automated classification according to the Minnesota code, including serial comparisons.[18,20-22] All ECG results were verified by visual inspection.

Identification and Classification of End Points

At each follow-up visit, adverse events were documented on the basis of the subjects' recall, and if appropriate, further information was

obtained from hospital records. All data on randomized subjects were flagged electronically on national computer data bases so that the numbers of deaths, incident cancers, hospitalizations, and cardiac surgeries could be monitored according to previously described methods.[23] Potential end points were reviewed and classified according to predefined criteria[16] by the End-Points Committee, whereas non–coronary heart disease events were reviewed and classified by the Adverse-Events Committee. The progress and conduct of the study were monitored regularly by the independent, unblinded Data and Safety Monitoring Committee. Except for the trial statistician and his assistant, all trial personnel remained unaware of the subjects' treatment assignments throughout the study.

Statistical Analysis

All data were analyzed according to the intention-to-treat principle. The results of the two fasting lipoprotein profiles obtained during visits 2 and 3 were averaged to produce base-line values. The LDL cholesterol results were analyzed according to both the treatment actually received and the intention-to-treat principle. The analysis based on actual treatment used only the measured lipid levels in subjects who had attended the previous scheduled visit and who had been issued with trial medication at that visit. For the intention-to-treat analysis, all recorded levels were included, without reference to the subjects' degree of compliance at previous visits. In addition, in cases in which no lipid value was available for a scheduled visit and no medication had been issued at the previous visit, the subject's base-line level was used. For each end-point category, the lengths of time to a first event were compared with use of the log-rank test, and the relative reduction in risk resulting from pravastatin treatment, with 95 percent confidence intervals, was calculated with the Cox proportional-hazards model.[24] In addition, Kaplan–Meier time-to-event curves were used to estimate the absolute risk of each event at five years for each treatment group. When a silent myocardial infarction was detected on the basis of serial comparison of ECGs, the event was con-

Table 1. Base-Line Characteristics of the Randomized Subjects, According to Treatment Group.*

CHARACTERISTIC	PLACEBO (N = 3293)	PRAVASTATIN (N = 3302)
Continuous variables		
Age — yr	55.1±5.5	55.3±5.5
Body-mass index†	26.0±3.1	26.0±3.2
Blood pressure — mm Hg		
Systolic	136±17	135±18
Diastolic	84±10	84±11
Cholesterol — mg/dl		
Total	272±22	272±23
LDL	192±17	192±17
HDL	44±10	44±9
Triglycerides — mg/dl	164±68	162±70
Alcohol consumption — units/wk‡	11±13	12±14
Categorical variables — no. of subjects (%)		
Angina§	174 (5)	164 (5)
Intermittent claudication§	96 (3)	97 (3)
Diabetes	35 (1)	41 (1)
Hypertension (self-reported)	506 (15)	531 (16)
Minor ECG abnormality	259 (8)	275 (8)
Smoking status		
Never smoked	705 (21)	717 (22)
Exsmoker	1127 (34)	1138 (34)
Current smoker	1460 (44)	1445 (44)
Employment status		
Employed	2324 (71)	2330 (71)
Unemployed	459 (14)	430 (13)
Retired	338 (10)	330 (10)
Disabled	171 (5)	210 (6)

*Plus–minus values are means ±SD. To convert values for cholesterol to millimoles per liter, multiply by 0.026, and to convert values for triglycerides to millimoles per liter, multiply by 0.011.

†The weight in kilograms divided by the square of the height in meters.

‡A unit was defined as 1 measure (60 ml) of liquor, 1 glass (170 ml) of wine, or a half pint (300 ml) of beer.

§As indicated by positive responses on the Rose questionnaire.

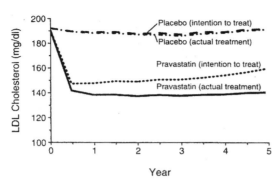

Figure 1. Effects of Pravastatin Therapy on Plasma LDL Cholesterol Levels.
To convert values for cholesterol to millimoles per liter, multiply by 0.026.

sidered to have occurred midway between the first diagnostic ECG and the previous ECG. Two-tailed P values were used throughout.

For the primary end point, an analysis was performed for predefined subgroups[18] characterized at base line according to age (<55 years or ≥55 years), smoking status (smoker or nonsmoker of cigarettes, cigars, or pipes), and whether at least two of the following risk factors were present: smoking, hypertension, a history of chest pain or intermittent claudication (as indicated by positive responses on the Rose questionnaire), diabetes, and a minor ECG abnormality associated with coronary heart disease (Minnesota code 4-2, 4-3, 5-2, or 5-3).

In addition, the effect of treatment was examined in a subgroup with and a subgroup without vascular disease at base line. Vascular disease was considered to be present if there was evidence of angina, intermittent claudication, stroke, transient ischemic attack, and ECG abnormalities according to the Minnesota code. Finally, the influence of base-line lipid levels on the effect of treatment was assessed by dividing the randomized population according to the median plasma cholesterol, LDL or HDL cholesterol, or plasma triglyceride concentration.

The Data and Safety Monitoring Committee conducted annual reviews of the main end points according to the O'Brien and Fleming criteria for stopping the trial prematurely.[25] The overall P value indicating statistical significance was set at 0.01.

RESULTS

A total of 6595 subjects underwent randomization. The clinical characteristics of the subjects who were screened and those who were randomized have been described previously.[26] The first patient was enrolled on February 1, 1989, and recruitment was completed by September 30, 1991. The final visits were made between February and May 1995, by which time the study population had accrued 32,216 subject-years of follow-up (an average of 4.9 years per subject). At the end of the study, the vital and clinical status of all randomized subjects was ascertained.

The base-line characteristics of the pravastatin and placebo groups are summarized in Table 1. As expected in a trial of this size, the groups were well balanced. For the study population as a whole, the average (±SD) plasma cholesterol level was 272±23 mg per deciliter (7.0±0.6 mmol per liter), the LDL cholesterol level was 192±17 mg per deciliter (5.0±0.5 mmol per liter), and the HDL cholesterol level was 44±9 mg per deciliter (1.14±0.26 mmol per liter). On the basis of positive responses on the Rose questionnaire, evidence of angina was present in 5 percent of the men, whereas 8 percent had ECG ST-T wave changes (Minnesota codes 4-2, 4-3, 5-2, and 5-3). The prevalence of self-reported diabetes mellitus was 1 percent, and that of hypertension was 16 percent; 44 percent of the subjects were current smokers.

Withdrawals

The cumulative rates of withdrawal from treatment in the placebo and pravastatin groups were 14.9 percent and 15.5 percent, respectively, at year 1, 19.1 percent and 19.4 percent at year 2, 22.5 percent and 22.7 percent at year 3, 25.2 percent and 24.7 percent at year 4, and 30.8 percent and 29.6 percent at year 5. There was no significant difference in the withdrawal rates between the two groups at any time. The disproportionate increase from year 4 to year 5 can be attributed to the withdrawal from the study of some subjects who had

Table 2. End Points of the Study.*

VARIABLE	PLACEBO (N = 3293)	PRAVASTATIN (N = 3302)	P VALUE	RISK REDUCTION WITH PRAVASTATIN (95% CI)
	no. of events (absolute % risk at 5 yr)			%
Definite coronary events				
Nonfatal MI or death from CHD	248 (7.9)	174 (5.5)	<0.001	31 (17 to 43)
Nonfatal MI (silent MIs omitted) or death from CHD	218 (7.0)	150 (4.7)	<0.001	33 (17 to 45)
Nonfatal MI	204 (6.5)	143 (4.6)	<0.001	31 (15 to 45)
Death from CHD	52 (1.7)	38 (1.2)	0.13	28 (−10 to 52)
Definite + suspected coronary events				
Nonfatal MI or death from CHD	295 (9.3)	215 (6.8)	<0.001	29 (15 to 40)
Nonfatal MI (silent MIs omitted) or death from CHD	240 (7.6)	166 (5.3)	<0.001	32 (17 to 44)
Nonfatal MI	246 (7.8)	182 (5.8)	0.001	27 (12 to 40)
Death from CHD	61 (1.9)	41 (1.3)	0.042	33 (1 to 55)
Other events				
Coronary angiography	128 (4.2)	90 (2.8)	0.007	31 (10 to 47)
PTCA or CABG	80 (2.5)	51 (1.7)	0.009	37 (11 to 56)
Fatal or nonfatal stroke	51 (1.6)	46 (1.6)	0.57	11 (−33 to 40)
Incident cancer	106 (3.3)	116 (3.7)	0.55	−8 (−41 to 17)
Death from other causes				
Other cardiovascular causes (including stroke)	12	9	—	—
Suicide	1	2	—	—
Trauma	5	3	—	—
Cancer	49 (1.5)	44 (1.3)	0.56	11 (−33 to 41)
All other causes	7	7	—	—
Death from all cardiovascular causes	73 (2.3)	50 (1.6)	0.033	32 (3 to 53)
Death from noncardiovascular causes	62 (1.9)	56 (1.7)	0.54	11 (−28 to 38)
Death from any cause	135 (4.1)	106 (3.2)	0.051	22 (0 to 40)

*The P values are based on the log-rank test. No formal analysis was carried out for events with a low incidence. CI denotes confidence interval. CHD coronary heart disease. MI myocardial infarction. PTCA percutaneous transluminal coronary angioplasty, and CABG coronary-artery bypass graft.

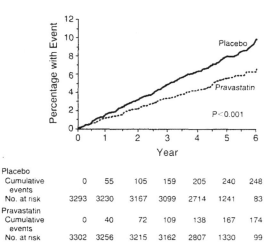

Placebo
| Cumulative events | 0 | 55 | 105 | 159 | 205 | 240 | 248 |
| No. at risk | 3293 | 3230 | 3167 | 3099 | 2714 | 1241 | 83 |

Pravastatin
| Cumulative events | 0 | 40 | 72 | 109 | 138 | 167 | 174 |
| No. at risk | 3302 | 3256 | 3215 | 3162 | 2807 | 1330 | 99 |

Figure 2. Kaplan–Meier Analysis of the Time to a Definite Non-fatal Myocardial Infarction or Death from Coronary Heart Disease, According to Treatment Group.

completed the five years of follow-up and who could have proceeded further but did not wish to do so.

Reduction in Lipid Levels

When the data were analyzed according to the treatment actually received, pravastatin was found to have lowered plasma levels of cholesterol by 20 percent, LDL cholesterol by 26 percent (Fig. 1), and triglycerides by 12 percent, whereas HDL cholesterol was increased by 5 percent. There were no such changes with placebo. When the data were analyzed according to the intention-to-treat principle, because such analysis includes subjects who withdrew and noncompliant subjects,

there was an apparent reduction in the observed difference in LDL cholesterol levels between treatment groups over time. This result is in contrast to that based on actual treatment, which showed that the difference was maintained.

End Points

As compared with placebo, pravastatin produced a significant reduction in the risk of the combined primary end point of definite nonfatal myocardial infarction and death from coronary heart disease (reduction, 31 percent; 95 percent confidence interval, 17 to 43 percent: P<0.001; absolute difference in the risk at five years, 2.4 percentage points) (Table 2 and Fig. 2). The effects of pravastatin on other principal end points are given in Table 2 and Figure 3. The reduction in the risk of nonfatal myocardial infarction was significant (P≤0.001) whether the definite cases of myocardial infarction were considered alone or in combination with suspected cases. Excluding silent myocardial infarctions from the analysis of the primary end point did not affect the outcome (Table 2). For the end point of death from coronary heart disease, there was a significant treatment effect in the analysis of both definite and suspected cases (risk reduction, 33 percent; 95 percent confidence interval, 1 to 55 percent; P = 0.042), but not in the analysis of definite cases alone, probably because of the smaller number of events in this group. However, there was a similar reduction in risk (28 percent). When the effect of treatment with pravastatin on death from all cardiovascular causes was analyzed, a 32 percent reduction in risk (95 percent confidence interval, 3 to 55 percent; P = 0.033) was observed. Treatment with pravastatin was associated with similar reductions in the frequency of coronary angiography (31 percent; 95 percent confidence interval, 10 to 47 percent; P = 0.007)

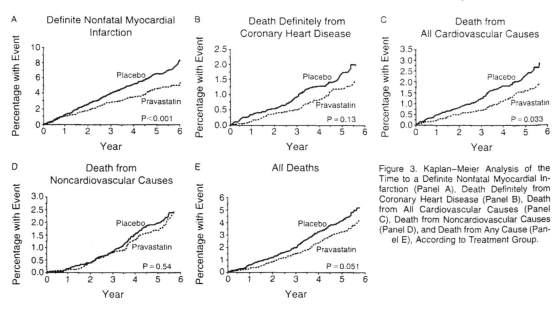

Figure 3. Kaplan–Meier Analysis of the Time to a Definite Nonfatal Myocardial Infarction (Panel A), Death Definitely from Coronary Heart Disease (Panel B), Death from All Cardiovascular Causes (Panel C), Death from Noncardiovascular Causes (Panel D), and Death from Any Cause (Panel E), According to Treatment Group.

and revascularization procedures (37 percent; 95 percent confidence interval, 11 to 56 percent; P = 0.009).

There were 56 deaths from noncardiovascular causes in the pravastatin group and 62 in the placebo group (P = 0.54). There was no significant difference between treatment groups in the numbers of deaths from cancer, suicide, or trauma. There were 46 strokes (6 of which were fatal) in the pravastatin group and 51 (4 fatal) in the placebo group. In the pravastatin group, the reduction in the number of deaths from cardiovascular causes in the absence of any increase in the number of deaths from noncardiovascular causes resulted in a 22 percent reduction in the overall risk of death (95 percent confidence interval, 0 to 40 percent; P = 0.051).

The beneficial effects of pravastatin therapy were evident in all subgroups (Table 3). The numbers of subjects in the subgroups with either multiple risk factors at base line or vascular disease at base line were too small to show a statistically significant effect.

Other Adverse Events

In the pravastatin group 116 subjects had incident (fatal or nonfatal) cancers, as compared with 106 in the placebo group (P = 0.55). These figures include cases of malignant melanoma but not minor skin cancers. For the placebo and pravastatin groups, respectively, there were 30 and 31 gastrointestinal cancers, 26 and 32 genitourinary cancers, 28 and 27 respiratory tract cancers, and 22 and 26 other cancers. Twenty subjects in the pravastatin group reported myalgia, and 97 muscle aches. The corresponding numbers in the placebo group were 19 and 102 (P not significant). Four subjects (three in the pravastatin group and one in the placebo group) had asymptomatic episodes of elevated creatine kinase concentrations (>10 times the upper reference limit). Elevations in aspartate aminotransferase and alanine aminotransferase values (>3 times the upper reference limits) were recorded for 26 and 16 subjects, respectively, in the pravastatin group, as compared with 20 and 12 subjects in the placebo group (P not significant).

DISCUSSION

As compared with placebo, pravastatin reduced the risk of fatal or nonfatal coronary events in middle-aged men with hypercholesterolemia and no history of myocardial infarction by approximately 30 percent. The beneficial effects of treatment were remarkably consistent across a variety of coronary end points. In contrast to the results of studies using resins, fibrates, or other

Table 3. Incidence of the Primary End Point, According to Subgroup.

VARIABLE	SUBGROUP	NO. OF SUBJECTS	PLACEBO	PRAVASTATIN	P VALUE*	RISK REDUCTION WITH PRAVASTATIN (95% CI)
			no. of events (absolute % risk at 5 yr)			*%*
Age	<55 yr	3225	96 (6.1)	57 (3.5)	0.0024	40 (16 to 56)
	≥55 yr	3370	152 (9.8)	117 (7.3)	0.0089	27 (8 to 43)
Current smoking status	Nonsmoker	3687	104 (6.0)	74 (4.3)	0.016	31 (6 to 48)
	Smoker	2905	144 (10.4)	100 (7.0)	0.0035	31 (12 to 47)
Multiple risk factors†	Absent	5401	178 (6.9)	114 (4.4)	<0.001	37 (20 to 50)
	Present	1194	70 (12.7)	60 (10.2)	0.20	20 (−13 to 43)
Cholesterol level‡	<269 mg/dl	3192	122 (8.1)	80 (5.4)	0.0019	36 (15 to 51)
	≥269 mg/dl	3403	126 (7.8)	94 (5.6)	0.021	27 (4 to 44)
LDL cholesterol level‡	<189 mg/dl	3211	110 (7.6)	71 (4.9)	0.0025	37 (15 to 53)
	≥189 mg/dl	3384	138 (8.3)	103 (6.1)	0.016	27 (6 to 43)
HDL cholesterol level‡	≥43 mg/dl	3304	99 (6.2)	66 (4.3)	0.011	33 (9 to 51)
	<43 mg/dl	3291	149 (9.7)	108 (6.7)	0.0035	31 (11 to 46)
Triglyceride level§	<148 mg/dl	3239	98 (6.3)	72 (4.4)	0.024	29 (4 to 48)
	≥148 mg/dl	3356	150 (9.4)	102 (6.6)	0.0025	32 (12 to 47)
Prior vascular disease	Absent	5529	183 (7.0)	125 (4.7)	<0.001	33 (15 to 46)
	Present	1066	65 (12.8)	49 (9.6)	0.075	29 (−4 to 51)

*The P values are based on the log-rank test.

†The presence of two or more of the following risk factors: smoking, hypertension, a history of chest pain or intermittent claudication (as indicated by positive responses on the Rose questionnaire), diabetes, and a minor ECG abnormality associated with coronary heart disease (Minnesota code 4-2, 4-3, 5-2, or 5-3).

‡To convert values for cholesterol to millimoles per liter, multiply by 0.026.

§To convert values for triglycerides to millimoles per liter, multiply by 0.011.

3-hydroxy-3-methylglutaryl–coenzyme A reductase inhibitors,[1-4,9] the time-to-event curves began to diverge within six months of the initiation of treatment and continued to do so at the same rate throughout the trial. The frequency of the need for coronary angiography and revascularization procedures was significantly lower in the pravastatin group than in the placebo group.

The subjects in this study were representative of the general population in terms of socioeconomic status and risk factors (Table 1). Their plasma cholesterol levels were in the highest quartile of the range found in the British population.[27] A number had evidence of minor vascular disease, and in order to make the findings of the trial applicable to typical middle-aged men with hypercholesterolemia, they were not excluded.

In line with accepted guidelines,[28] the LDL cholesterol level was used as a criterion for entry into the study. As compared with placebo, pravastatin produced a major reduction in this lipoprotein fraction (Fig. 1) and moderate decreases in plasma triglycerides, as well as an increase in HDL cholesterol. These changes are in line with the expected response to pravastatin,[29] and all could potentially result in clinical benefit. The changes in the LDL cholesterol level are more substantial than those observed in earlier primary prevention studies.[1-4]

When the subjects were divided into two groups according to their lipid levels at base line, we found that coronary risk was related to higher plasma LDL cholesterol and triglyceride levels (i.e., levels above the median values) and lower HDL cholesterol levels (i.e., levels below the median value) (Table 3). The plasma cholesterol level was not a significant factor, principally because of the narrow range of cholesterol values used as a criterion for entry into the study. The relative reduction in risk with pravastatin therapy was statistically significant and of a similar magnitude in subjects with lipid values above and below the median.

The relative reductions in risk attributable to pravastatin therapy were not affected by age (<55 years vs. ≥55 years) or smoking status. Furthermore, a significant treatment effect was seen in the subgroup without multiple risk factors and the subgroup without preexisting vascular disease. Thus, it is possible to conclude that in the subjects who might be considered to fall strictly into the primary-prevention category, pravastatin therapy produced a significant reduction in the relative risk of a coronary event.

Pravastatin therapy was well tolerated and resulted in no more study withdrawals than placebo. In particular, as in an earlier study,[15] there was no evidence that pravastatin adversely affected liver function or caused myopathy. Our results support those of a recent secondary-prevention trial[9] that found that lipid lowering with a 3-hydroxy-3-methylglutaryl–coenzyme A reductase inhibitor is not associated with an increased risk of death from noncardiovascular causes. As in that earlier trial,[9] a comparison of the treatment and placebo groups showed no significant increase in the incidence of fatal or incident cancers or deaths due to suicide or trauma. More data on the adverse-event profile of this class of drugs will become available as the results of other prevention trials are published. In the current study, the benefit of pravastatin therapy with respect to fatal coronary events and the absence of any increase in the number of deaths from other causes led to a 22 percent reduction in the relative risk of death from any cause (P = 0.051).

From the data in Table 2, it can be estimated that treating 1000 middle-aged men with hypercholesterolemia and no evidence of a previous myocardial infarction with pravastatin for five years will result in 14 fewer coronary angiograms, 8 fewer revascularization procedures, 20 fewer nonfatal myocardial infarctions, 7 fewer deaths from cardiovascular causes, and 2 fewer deaths from other causes than would be expected in the absence of treatment. Since these figures are based on an intention-to-treat analysis, the magnitude of the benefit in fully compliant subjects is likely to be greater. These findings can be compared favorably with the results of the Medical Research Council trial[30,31] of the treatment of mild hypertension in middle-aged subjects. In that study, it was estimated that five years of active treatment of 1000 men ranging in age from 35 to 64 years would result in six fewer strokes and two fewer cardiovascular events than would be expected. Thus, our results indicate that reducing cholesterol levels with pravastatin reduces the risk of coronary events in asymptomatic subjects with hypercholesterolemia.

APPENDIX

The members of the West of Scotland Coronary Prevention Study are as follows: *Executive Committee (Voting Members)* — J. Shepherd (chairman), S.M. Cobbe, A.R. Lorimer, J.H. McKillop, I. Ford, C.J. Packard, P.W. Macfarlane, and G.C. Isles; *Data and Safety Monitoring Committee* — M.F. Oliver (chairman), A.F. Lever, B.W. Brown, J.G.G. Ledingham, S.J. Pocock, and B.M. Rifkind; *End-Points Committee* — S.M. Cobbe, B.D. Vallance, P.W. Macfarlane; *Adverse-Events Committee* — A.R. Lorimer, J.H. McKillop, and D. Ballantyne; *Data-Center Staff* — L. Anderson, D. Duncan, J. McGrath, S. Kean, A. Lawrence, V. Montgomery, and J. Norrie; *Population Screening* — M. Percy; *Clinical Coordination, Monitoring, and Administration* — E. Pomphrey, A. Whitehouse, P. Cameron, P. Parker, F. Porteous, L. Fletcher, and C. Kilday; *Computerized ECG Analysis* — D. Shoat (deceased), S. Latif, and J. Kennedy; *Laboratory Operations* — M.A. Bell and R. Birrell; and *Company Liaison and General Support* — M. Mellies, J. Meyer, and W. Campbell.

REFERENCES

1. A co-operative trial in the primary prevention of ischaemic heart disease using clofibrate: report from the Committee of Principal Investigators. Br Heart J 1978;40:1069-118.
2. The Lipid Research Clinics Coronary Primary Prevention Trial results. I. Reduction in incidence of coronary heart disease. JAMA 1984;251:351-64.
3. The Lipid Research Clinics Coronary Primary Prevention Trial results. II. The relationship of reduction in incidence of coronary heart disease to cholesterol lowering. JAMA 1984;251:365-74.
4. Frick MH, Elo O, Haapa K, et al. Helsinki Heart Study: primary-prevention trial with gemfibrozil in middle-aged men with dyslipidemia: safety of treatment, changes in risk factors, and incidence of coronary heart disease. N Engl J Med 1987;317:1237-45.
5. Oliver MF. Might treatment of hypercholesterolaemia increase non-cardiac mortality? Lancet 1991;337:1529-31.
6. Hulley SB, Walsh JMB, Newman TB. Health policy on blood cholesterol: time to change directions. Circulation 1992;86:1026-9.
7. Davey Smith G, Pekkanen J. Should there be a moratorium on the use of cholesterol lowering drugs? BMJ 1992;304:431-4.
8. LaRosa JC, Hunninghake D, Bush D, et al. The cholesterol facts: a summary of the evidence relating dietary fats, serum cholesterol, and coronary heart disease: a joint statement by the American Heart Association and the National Heart, Lung, and Blood Institute. Circulation 1990;81:1721-33.
9. The Scandinavian Simvastatin Survival Study Group. Randomised trial of cholesterol lowering in 4444 patients with coronary heart disease: the Scandinavian Simvastatin Survival Study (4S). Lancet 1994;344:1383-9.
10. MAAS Investigators. Effect of simvastatin on coronary atheroma: the Multicentre Anti-Atheroma Study (MAAS). Lancet 1994;344:633-8. [Erratum, Lancet 1994;344:762.]
11. Furberg CD, Adams HP Jr, Applegate WB, et al. Effect of lovastatin on early carotid atherosclerosis and cardiovascular events. Circulation 1994;90:1679-87.
12. Jukema JW, Bruschke AVG, van Boven AJ, et al. Effects of lipid lowering by pravastatin on progression and regression of coronary artery disease in symptomatic men with normal to moderately elevated serum cholesterol levels: the Regression Growth Evaluation Statin Study (REGRESS). Circulation 1995;91:2528-40.
13. Crouse JR III, Byington RP, Bond MG, et al. Pravastatin, Lipids, and Atherosclerosis in the Carotid Arteries (PLAC-II). Am J Cardiol 1995;75:455-9. [Erratum, Am J Cardiol 1995;75:862.]
14. Pitt B, Mancini GBJ, Ellis SG, Rosman HS, Park J-SP, McGovern ME. Pravastatin Limitation of Atherosclerosis in the Coronary Arteries (PLAC I): reduction in atherosclerosis progression and clinical events. J Am Coll Cardiol (in press).
15. The Pravastatin Multinational Study Group for Cardiac Risk Patients. Effects of pravastatin in patients with serum total cholesterol levels from 5.2 to 7.8 mmol/liter (200 to 300 mg/dl) plus two additional atherosclerotic risk factors. Am J Cardiol 1993;72:1031-7.
16. West of Scotland Coronary Prevention Study Group. A coronary primary prevention study of Scottish men age 45-64 years: trial design. J Clin Epidemiol 1992;45:849-60.
17. EAS Task Force for Prevention of Coronary Heart Disease. Prevention of coronary heart disease: scientific background and new clinical guidelines. Nutr Metab Cardiovasc Dis 1992;2:113-56.
18. Prineas RJ, Crow RS, Blackburn H. The Minnesota code manual of electrocardiographic findings: standards and procedures for measurement and classification. Boston: John Wright, PSG, 1982.
19. Lipid Research Clinics manual of laboratory operations. 1975. Washington, D.C.: Government Printing Office, 1975. (DHEW publication no. (NIH) 85-268.)
20. Crow RS, Prineas RJ, Jacobs DR Jr, Blackburn H. A new epidemiologic classification system for interim myocardial infarction from serial electrocardiographic changes. Am J Cardiol 1989;64:454-61.

21. Macfarlane PW, Devine B, Latif S, McLaughlin S, Shoat DB, Watts MP. Methodology of ECG interpretation in the Glasgow program. Methods Inf Med 1990;29:354-61.

22. Macfarlane PW, Latif S, Shoat DS, Cobbe SM. Automated serial ECG comparison using the Minnesota Code. Eur Heart J 1990;11:Suppl:411. abstract.

23. West of Scotland Coronary Prevention Study Group. Computerised record linkage: compared with traditional follow-up methods in clinical trials and illustrated in a prospective epidemiologic study. J Clin Epidemiol (in press).

24. Collett D. Modelling survival data in medical research. London: Chapman & Hall, 1994.

25. O'Brien PC, Fleming TR. A multiple testing procedure for clinical trials. Biometrics 1979;35:549-56.

26. West of Scotland Coronary Prevention Study Group. Screening experience and baseline characteristics in the West of Scotland Coronary Prevention Study. Am J Cardiol 1995;76:485-91.

27. Mann JI, Lewis B, Shepherd J, et al. Blood lipid concentrations and other cardiovascular risk factors: distribution, prevalence, and detection in Britain. BMJ 1988;296:1702-6.

28. Summary of the second report of the National Cholesterol Education Program (NCEP) expert panel on detection, evaluation, and treatment of high blood cholesterol in adults (Adult Treatment Panel II). JAMA 1993;269:3015-23.

29. Jones PH, Farmer JA, Cressman MD, et al. Once-daily pravastatin in patients with primary hypercholesterolemia: a dose-response study. Clin Cardiol 1991;14:146-51.

30. Medical Research Council Working Party. MRC trial of treatment of mild hypertension: principal results. BMJ 1985;291:97-104.

31. Miall WE, Greenberg G. Mild hypertension: is there pressure to treat? An account of the MRC trial. Cambridge, United Kingdom: Cambridge University Press, 1987.

Citation:

Are the results of this single preventive or therapeutic trial valid?

Was the assignment of patients to treatments randomised?
Was the randomisation list concealed?

Were all patients who entered the trial accounted for at its conclusion?
Were they analysed in the groups to which they were randomised?

Were patients and clinicians kept 'blind' to which treatment was being received?

Aside from the experimental treatment, were the groups treated equally?

Were the groups similar at the start of the trial?

Are the valid results of this randomised trial important?

SAMPLE CALCULATIONS (see pp134–40 of *Evidence-based Medicine*).

Occurrence of diabetic neuropathy		Relative risk reduction (RRR)	Absolute risk reduction (ARR)	Number needed to treat (NNT)
Usual insulin control event rate (CER)	Intensive insulin experimental event rate (EER)	$\dfrac{CER - EER}{CER}$	$CER - EER$	$1/ARR$
9.6%	2.8%	$\dfrac{9.6\% - 2.8\%}{9.6\%}$ $= 71\%$	$9.6\% - 2.8\%$ $= 6.8\%$	$1/6.8\%$ $= 15$ pts

95% confidence interval (CI) on an NNT = 1 / (limits on the CI of its ARR) =

$$+/-1.96\sqrt{\frac{CER \times (1-CER)}{\#\text{ of control pts}} + \frac{EER \times (1-EER)}{\#\text{ of exper. pts}}} = +/-1.96\sqrt{\frac{0.096 \times 0.904}{730} + \frac{0.028 \times 0.972}{711}} = +/-2.4\%$$

Are the valid results of this randomised trial important?

YOUR CALCULATIONS

		Relative risk reduction (RRR)	Absolute risk reduction (ARR)	Number needed to treat (NNT)
CER	EER	$\dfrac{CER - EER}{CER}$	CER – EER	1/ARR

Can you apply this valid, important evidence about a treatment in caring for your patient?

Do these results apply to your patient?

Is your patient so different from those in the trial that its results can't help you?

How great would the potential benefit of therapy actually be for your individual patient?

Method I: **f**

Risk of the outcome in your patient, relative to patients in the trial.
Expressed as a decimal: _____
NNT/f = ____/____ =
_____
(NNT for patients like yours)

Method II: **1 / (PEER x RRR)**

Your patient's expected event rate if they received the control treatment: PEER:
1 / (PEER x RRR) = 1/_____ = _____
(NNT for patients like yours)

Are your patient's values and preferences satisfied by the regimen and its consequences?

Do your patient and you have a clear assessment of their values and preferences?

Are they met by this regimen and its consequences?

Additional notes

Citation: Shepherd J *et al.* (1995) Prevention of coronary heart disease with pravastatin in men with hypercholesterolemia. *NEJM.* **333**: 1301–7.

Are the results of this single preventive or therapeutic trial valid?

Was the assignment of patients to treatments randomised?	**Yes.**
Was the randomisation list concealed?	**Yes.**
Were all patients who entered the trial accounted for at its conclusion? Were they analysed in the groups to which they were randomised?	**Yes. The clinical and vital status of every participant was known at follow-up, and the study was analysed on the intention to treat principle.**
Were patients and clinicians kept 'blind' to which treatment was being received?	**Yes.**
Aside from the experimental treatment, were the groups treated equally?	**Yes.**
Were the groups similar at the start of the trial?	**Yes.**

Are the valid results of this randomised trial important?

SAMPLE CALCULATIONS (see pp134–40 of *Evidence-based Medicine*)

Occurrence of diabetic neuropathy		Relative risk reduction (RRR)	Absolute risk reduction (ARR)	Number needed to treat (NNT)
(CER)	(EER)	$\dfrac{\text{CER} - \text{EER}}{\text{CER}}$	CER − EER	1/ARR
9.6%	2.8%	$\dfrac{9.6\% - 2.8\%}{9.6\%}$ = 71%	9.6% − 2.8% = 6.8%	1/6.8% = 15 pts

95% confidence interval (CI) on an NNT = 1 / (limits on the CI of its ARR) =

$$+/-1.96\sqrt{\frac{\text{CER} \times (1-\text{CER})}{\text{\# of control pts}} + \frac{\text{EER} \times (1-\text{EER})}{\text{\# of exper. pts}}} = +/-1.96\sqrt{\frac{0.096 \times 0.904}{730} + \frac{0.028 \times 0.972}{711}} = +/-2.4\%$$

YOUR CALCULATIONS (for the outcome of non-fatal MI or death from CHD after five years)

CER	EER	Relative risk reduction (RRR)	Absolute risk reduction (ARR)	Number needed to treat (NNT)
		$\dfrac{\text{CER} - \text{EER}}{\text{CER}}$	CER – EER	1/ARR
7.5%	5.3%	$\dfrac{7.5\% - 5.3\%}{7.5\%}$ = 29% (14% to 45%)	7.5% – 5.3% = 2.2% (1% to 3.4%)	45 (30 to 98)

95% confidence interval (CI) on an NNT = 1 / (limits on the CI of its ARR) = +/– 1.2%

Can you apply this valid, important evidence about a treatment in caring for your patient?

Do these results apply to your patient?

Is your patient so different from those in the trial that its results can't help you?	**The trial was conducted in men aged 45–64, whereas our patient is a 44-year old woman. Clinical judgement required! Is there a good reason why the treatment should have different qualitative effects in men and women?**
How great would the potential benefit of therapy actually be for your individual patient?	To judge this we used the New Zealand tables (see notes below) to calculate an absolute risk of cardiovascular disease over the next five years for a woman with this risk factor profile. We adjusted her risk upwards one level to account for the family history of sudden death. This suggested a five year risk of 2.5–5%, about half that in the control group of the trial.
Method I: **f**	Risk of the outcome in your patient, relative to patients in the trial. Expressed as a decimal: • for fatal or non-fatal coronary event: NNT/f = **45/0.5 = 90** • for death from CHD the NNT is **250** and • NNT/f = **250/0.5 = 500** (NNT for patients like yours)
Method II: **1 / (PEER x RRR)**	Your patient's expected event rate if they received the control treatment: PEER: **4%** 1 / (PEER x RRR) = **1/.012 = 83** (NNT for patients like yours)
Are your patient's values and preferences satisfied by the regimen and its consequences?	**This will require discussion with the patient. Her absolute risk of having a myocardial infarction is quite low and she will only reduce her absolute risk by about 1% from taking drug treatment. Her risk of dying from coronary disease is smaller still. She may wish instead to reconsider lifestyle change and agree a follow-up programme with you.**
Do your patient and you have a clear assessment of their values and preferences?	**For discussion. The relatively high cost of the drug and the high NNT will be factors for the doctor and patient to consider.**
Are they met by this regimen and its consequences?	**Needs to be addressed in each patient.**

Additional notes

1 Based on prognostic data from the Framingham Study, the New Zealand tables allow the calculation of an absolute risk of cardiovascular disease based on gender, age, smoking history, presence or absence of diabetes, blood pressure and Cholesterol:HDL cholesterol ratio. By courtesy of Dr Rod Jackson, they can be accessed on the internet at: http://cebm.jr2.ox.ac.uk/docs/prognosis.html
2 The parents need to be evaluated. They have established vascular disease and therefore face a high absolute risk of further cardiovascular events. The NNT for cholesterol lowering would be much lower for them.

CAT – EFFECTIVENESS OF PRAVASTATIN FOR PRIMARY PREVENTION OF CARDIOVASCULAR DISEASE

Clinical Bottom Line

Pravastatin reduced the risk of definite coronary events (non-fatal MI or death from CHD) in asymptomatic middle-aged men. Reductions in coronary deaths were not statisistically significant. The NNTs are high as the absolute risk was low, and would be lower still for our patient.

Citation

Shepherd J, Cobbe SM, Ford I *et al.* (1995) Prevention of coronary heart disease with pravastatin in men with hypercholesterolemia. West of Scotland Coronary Prevention Study Group. *NEJM.* **333:** 1301–7.

Clinical Question

In a 44-year old woman without a history of cardiovascular disease, does lowering cholesterol with drug treatment lead to a reduction in the risk of myocardial infarction?

Search Terms

'cholesterol' and 'drug' in *Best Evidence.*

The Study

6995 men, aged 45 to 64, with no history of myocardial infarction, were recruited from screening clinics in Scotland if they had evidence of hypercholesterolaemia (cholesterol >6.5 mmol/L which did not reduce signficantly with eight weeks of dietary advice). Their mean plasma cholesterol at baseline was 7.0 mmol/L. They were randomised to receive 40 mg of pravastatin or placebo and followed for up to five years. Medical records, ECG recordings, and the national death registry were used to determine the clinical endpoints, and there was complete ascertainment of the endpoints.

The Evidence

Outcome	Time to outcome	CER	EER	RRR	ARR	NNT
Non-fatal MI or death from CHD	5 years	0.075	0.053	29%	0.022	45
95% confidence intervals				14% to 45%	0.010 to 0.034	30 to 98
Death from CHD	5 years	0.016	0.012	25%	0.004	250
95% confidence intervals				−10% to 60%	−0.002 to 0.010	NNT = 103 to Inf NNH = 598 to Inf
Death from all cardiovascular causes	5 years	0.022	0.015	32%	0.007	143
95% confidence intervals				2% to 61%	0.000 to 0.014	74 to 2012

Outcome	PEER	NNT (PEER)	F	NNT (f)
Non-fatal MI or death from CHD			.5	90
Death from CHD			.5	500
Death from all cardiovascular causes			.5	286

Comments

1 The trial was conducted in men aged 45–64. Our patient is a 44-year old woman. We need to make a decision about whether the qualitative effects of cholesterol lowering are likely to be the same in men and women.

2 If we accept that the relative effects are the same, we have to take into account our patient's baseline risk in deciding the magnitude of the benefits she might expect from the treatment.

3 The rates and risk reductions calculated here differ slightly from those given in the paper, because the authors used survival analysis in determining absolute risk at five years.

Your turn: case-presentations

- Take one of your patients who presented an important problem in therapy, diagnosis, prognosis or harm.

- Formulate that problem into a three-part question (the patient, the manoeuvre and the outcome), based on what you learn from Session 1.

- Do a search for the best evidence based on what you learn from Sessions 3-5 (lots of help available from us or the library team).

- Critically appraise that evidence for its validity, importance, and usefulness.

- Integrate that appraisal with clinical expertise and summarise it (in a 1-pager if you wish).

- Present it to the rest of us at one of the final sessions. (Certificates will be given to presenters.)

PART A Critical appraisal of a clinical article about diagnosis

During a long night on call, you are twice asked to visit children under the age of ten, whose parents have told you that their child is 'burning up'. In the first case, the 5-year old child has symptoms of a cold and the temperature is normal when you measure it. The second child, a 2-year old, appears much more ill, the recorded temperature is 39.5. After examining the child, you are concerned there may be serious illness, and refer the child to hospital where a diagnosis of urinary tract infection is confirmed.

Over coffee the next morning, you discuss the two different outcomes and wonder whether a parent's description of a child 'burning up' has any diagnostic value. Your curiosity is further whetted when one of your partners comments that he does not carry a thermometer on call, because 'the back of your hand is all you need'. You form the clinical question: 'In the diagnosis of fever in children is palpation, by mother or doctor, accurate in comparison to recording the temperature with a thermometer?'

You perform a MEDLINE search using the free text term 'fever' and the MeSH terms ('sensitivity and specificity') and find a short paper on diagnosing fever using touch. This is readily available in the practice library: *BMJ* (1998) **317:** 321.

Read this article and decide:
1   Are the results of this diagnostic article valid?
2   Are the valid results of this diagnostic study important?
3   Can you apply this valid, important evidence about a diagnostic test in caring for your patient?

If you want to read some strategies for answering these sorts of questions, you could have a look at pp 81–4, 118–28 and 159–63 in *Evidence-based Medicine.*

PART B Introduction to the CATMaker (optional)

We will give you a copy of the CATMaker and show you how to use it to generate and save your own one-page 'Critically Appraised Topic (CAT)' from an article about therapy. The advantages of the CATMaker include its ability to calculate for you the clinically useful measures of the effects of therapy and their confidence intervals, and to save your critical appraisal for printing, sharing and storage.

Now would be a good time to start searching on potential topics for your presentations in Sessions 6 and 7!

2 Bruce M, Will RG, Ironside JW, McConnell I, Drummond D, Suttie A, et al. Transmissions to mice indicate that 'new variant' CJD is caused by the BSE agent. *Nature* 1997;389:498-501.
3 Hill AF, Desbruslais M, Joiner S, Sidle KCL, Gowland I, Collinge J, et al. The same prion strain causes vCJD and BSE. *Nature* 1997;389:448-50.

4 Homer AC, Honavar M, Lantos PL, Hastie IR, Kellett JM, Millard PH. Diagnosing dementia: do we get it right? *BMJ* 1988;297:894-6.
5 Cousens SN, Vynnycky E, Zeidler M, Will RG, Smith PG. Predicting the CJD epidemic in humans. *Nature* 1997;385:197-8.

(Accepted 6 March 1998)

Diagnosing fever by touch: observational study

Katherine Whybrew, Matthew Murray, Colin Morley

Fever is a useful indicator of whether a child is seriously ill.[1] Many mothers and doctors estimate children's temperature by touch.[2] We assessed whether mothers and medical students could use touch to determine if children had fever.

Subjects, methods, and results

During their elective in a Zambian hospital, medical students and the child's mother felt children's abdomen, forehead, and neck and independently recorded whether the child felt hot. Simultaneously, a mercury thermometer was used to measure axillary temperature for exactly 3 minutes. Rectal temperature measurement was not permitted at this hospital.

In total, 1090 children aged 1 month to 16 years (median 2 years) were studied. The mean ambient temperature was 24.5 (SD 2.0)°C; the mean axillary temperature from 24 children not recently vaccinated and with no complaint was 36.7 (2SD 1.12)°C. Therefore 37.8°C or higher was defined as a fever. With this definition, 236 (27%) children had fever.

The mothers assessed 862 children and thought 574 (67%) were warm or hot. Their sensitivity was 94% (221/236), specificity 44% (273/626), positive predictive value 39% (221/574), and negative predictive value 95% (273/288).

Two students assessed 1086 children and thought 525 (48%) were warm or hot. Their sensitivity was 94% (257/274), specificity 67% (544/812), positive predictive value 49% (257/525), and negative predictive value 97% (544/561). Two students, working independently, had remarkably similar results (sensitivities 95% and 94%, positive predictive values 50% and 47%). The table shows the data for the two groups:

Comment

This study showed that when mothers and medical students felt the children they rarely missed a child with fever, but they overestimated the number who had fever.

Because it was impractical to measure rectal temperature for cultural reasons, axillary temperature had to be used. Axillary temperature is not always accurate. One study comparing axillary and rectal temperature found means of 36.8°C and 37.4°C, respectively, and a median difference of 0.5°C (range −1.0°C to 3.2°C).[3] The difference was largest in children with high fever. The shortcomings of axillary temperature measurement might have influenced our results: positive predictive values might have been higher if rectal temperature been used.

These children felt warmer than did children in Britain, possibly because of the higher ambient temperature and the tendency to overdress. Therefore, rather than use a range derived from a different population, we calculated a normal range for the group. Defining fever as a temperature of 37.8°C or more was higher than the temperature used in other studies (37.2°C,[3] 37.4°C,[4] and 37.5°C[5]). In our study the thermometer was assiduously kept in the axilla for 3 minutes. In other studies the temperature was taken for a shorter time, which may account for the lower temperatures used.

A recent African study investigated the ability of patients (1606 men and children) or their carers to decide whether they had a fever.[5] Twenty per cent had fever, but only 28% of those thought to have fever did; of those thought to have a normal temperature, 92% did.

These two studies establish that, as a screening procedure, touch will seriously overestimate the incidence of fever, but with touch, fever will rarely be missed; also, a patient who does not feel hot is very likely not to have fever. A child who feels hot needs to have a temperature taken before fever is diagnosed.

Thanks to the parents and children who took part in the study and the helpful staff of Chikankata Hospital, Zambia.

Contributors: KW and MM collected the data and were closely involved in data analysis and presentation. CM suggested the project, helped with data analysis and presentation, and is guarantor for the paper.

Funding: Financial assistance from the Commonwealth Foundation; Churchill College, Cambridge; Pembroke College, Cambridge; Medical Defence Union; Lady Valerie France; John Zeal.

Conflict of interest: None.

University of Cambridge, Department of Paediatrics, Box 226 Neonatal Intensive Care Unit, Addenbrooke's Hospital, Cambridge CB2 2QQ
Katherine Whybrew, *medical student*
Matthew Murray, *medical student*
Colin Morley, *honorary consultant paediatrician*

Correspondence to: Dr Morley morleyc@cryptic.rch.unimelb.edu.au

BMJ 1998;317:321

1 Morley CJ, Thornton AJ, Cole TJ, Hewson PH, Fowler A. Baby Check: a scoring system to grade the severity of acute systemic illness in babies under 6 months old. *Arch Dis Child* 1991;66:100-5.
2 Clarke S. Use of thermometers in general practice. *BMJ* 1992;304:961-3.
3 Morley CJ, Hewson PH, Thornton AJ, Cole TJ. Axillary and rectal temperature. *Arch Dis Child* 1992;67:122-5.
4 Shann F, MacKenzie A. Comparison of rectal, axillary and forehead temperatures. *Arch Ped Adolesc Med* 1996;150:74-8.
5 Einterz EM, Bates ME. Fever in Africa: do patients know when they are hot? *Lancet* 1997;350:781.

(Accepted 2 February 1998)

Determination of fever in children by mothers and medical students and by axillary temperature ≥37.8°C

	Axillary temperature		
	≥37.8°C	<37.8°C	Total
Mothers:	236	626	862
Child feels warm or hot	221	353	574
Child feels normal or cold	15	273	288
Students:	274	812	1086
Child feels warm or hot	257	268	525
Child feels normal or cold	17	544	561

Session 2 – Diagnosis & introduction to the CATMaker software

Citation:

Are the results of this diagnostic study valid?

Was there an independent, blind comparison with a
reference ('gold') standard of diagnosis?

Was the diagnostic test evaluated in an appropriate
spectrum of patients (like those in whom it would
be used in practice)?

Was the reference standard applied regardless of
the diagnostic test result?

Are the valid results of this diagnostic study important?

SAMPLE CALCULATIONS (see p120 of *Evidence-based Medicine*)

		Target disorder (iron deficiency anaemia)		Totals
		Present	**Absent**	
Diagnostic test result	Positive (<65 mmol/L)	731 a	270 b	a+b 1001
(serum ferritin)	Negative (≥65 mmol/L)	78 c	1500 d	c+d 1578
	Totals	809 a+c	1770 b+d	a+b+c+d 2579

Sensitivity = a/(a+c) = 731/809 = 90%

Specificity = d/(b+d) = 1500/1770 = 85%

Likelihood Ratio for a positive test result = LR+ = sens/(1–spec) = 90%/15% = 6

Likelihood Ratio for a negative test result = LR– = (1–sens)/spec = 10%/85% = 0.12

Positive Predictive Value = a/(a+b) = 731/1001 = 73%

Negative Predictive Value = d/(c+d) = 1500/1578 = 95%

Pre-test Probability (prevalence) = (a+c)/(a+b+c+d) = 809/2579 = 32%

Pre-test-odds = prevalence/(1–prevalence) = 31%/69% = 0.45

Post-test odds = Pre-test odds x Likelihood Ratio

Post-test Probability = Post-test odds/(Post-test odds + 1)

Are the valid results of this diagnostic study important?

YOUR CALCULATIONS

		Target disorder		Totals
		Present	**Absent**	
Diagnostic test result	Positive	a	b	a+b
	Negative	c	d	c+d
	Totals	a+c	b+d	a+b+c+d

Sensitivity = a/(a+c) =   Specificity = d/(b+d) =

Likelihood Ratio for a positive test result = LR+ = sens/(1–spec) =

Likelihood Ratio for a negative test result = LR– = (1–sens)/spec =

Positive Predictive Value = a/(a+b) =   Negative Predictive Value = d/(c+d) =

Pre-test Probability (prevalence) = (a+c)/(a+b+c+d) =

Pre-test-odds = prevalence/(1–prevalence) =

Post-test odds = Pre-test odds x Likelihood Ratio =

Post-test Probability = Post-test odds/(Post-test odds + 1) =

Can you apply this valid, important evidence about a diagnostic test in caring for your patient?

Is the diagnostic test available, affordable, accurate, and precise in your setting?	
Can you generate a clinically sensible estimate of your patient's pre-test probability (from practice data, personal experience, the report itself, or clinical speculation).	
Will the resulting post-test probabilities affect your management and help your patient? (Could it move you across a test-treatment threshold? Would your patient be a willing partner in carrying it out?)	
Would the consequences of the test help your patient?	

Additional notes

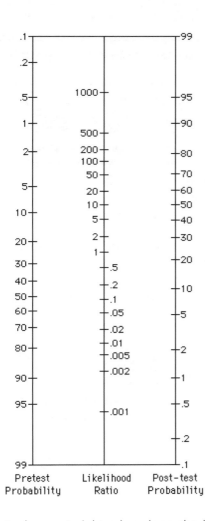

Anchor a straight-edge along the left edge of the nomogram at your patient's pre-test probability and pivot it until it intersects the likelihood ratio for your patent's diagnostic test result. It will intersect the right edge of the nomogram at your patient's post-test probability. Test 1: for a likelihood ratio of 1, pre-test and post-test probabilities should be identical. Test 2: for a pre-test probability of 30% and a likelihood ratio of 5, the post-test probability is just under 70%.

Adapted from Fagan TJ (1975) Nomogram for Bayes' theorem. *N Engl J Med*. **293:** 257.

> Citation: Whybrew K, Murray M, Morley C (1998) Diagnosing fever by touch: observational study. *BMJ.* **317**: 321.

Are the results of this diagnostic study valid?

Was there an independent, blind comparison with a reference ('gold') standard of diagnosis?	**Yes, all patients had an axillary temperature measured for three minutes, although it was not clear if the assessor was blind to the results of touching the patient.**
Was the diagnostic test evaluated in an appropriate spectrum of patients (like those in whom it would be used in practice)?	**Yes, although few details about the population are provided in this paper.**
Was the reference standard applied regardless of the diagnostic test result?	**Yes.**

Are the valid results of this diagnostic study important?

Sensitivity, specificity and predictive value have been calculated by the authors. We calculated the following likelihood ratios according to whether the examiner was the mother or a medical student:

	Temperature >37.8	Temperature <37.8	Likelihood ratio
Mother feels:			
Child warm or hot	221	353	1.7
Child normal or cold	15	273	0.14
Students feel:			
Child warm or hot	257	268	2.8
Child normal or cold	17	544	0.09

- **For pre-test probablities in the 30–70% range, a mother's judgement that the child is hot yields post-test probabilities of 40–75%. A medical student's assessment yields post-test probablities of 65–90%. So in most cases, a positive test is not going to change the probabilities enough to make it a helpful test.**

- **For pre-test probabilities in the 30–70% range, a mother's judgement that the child is not hot yields post-test probabilities of 4–20%, and a medical student's judgement yields post-test probabilites of 3–10%. So, in a child in whom there are no other signs to suggest infection is present, if the child feels cool, a temperature is unlikely to be present (a SnNouT).**

- **Diagnosing fever by touch is a helpful clinical measurement if the child feels cool. It is less helpful when the child feels hot, because many of these children in fact have normal temperatures.**

Can you apply this valid, important evidence about a diagnostic test in caring for your patient?

Is the diagnostic test available, affordable, accurate and precise in your setting?	**In this case, the diagnostic test is a simple clinical finding and is free and readily available.**
Can you generate a clinically sensible estimate of your patient's pre-test probability (from practice data, from personal experience, from the report itself, or from clinical speculation).	**In deciding the probability of serious infection, we need to take into account a number of other factors in the history and examination.**
Will the resulting post-test probabilities affect your management and help your patient? (Could it move you across a test-treatment threshold? Would your patient be a willing partner in carrying it out?)	**Asking mothers to record a temperature when they feel the child is warm might allow you to provide reassurance over the phone (and avoid a visit), if there are no other worrying features in the history. Your partner who thinks he doesn't need to carry a thermometer is right if the child feels cool, but he will over-diagnose fever if he judges that all children who feel hot have temperatures.**

Additional notes

A LIKELIHOOD RATIO NOMOGRAM

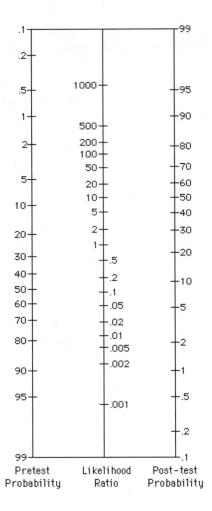

Anchor a straight-edge along the left edge of the nomogram at your patient's pre-test probability and pivot it until it intersects the likelihood ratio for your patent's diagnostic test result. It will intersect the right edge of the nomogram at your patient's post-test probability. Test 1: for a likelihood ratio of 1, pre-test and post-test probabilities should be identical. Test 2: for a pre-test probability of 30% and a likelihood ratio of 5, the post-test probability is just under 70%.

Adapted from Fagan TJ (1975) Nomogram for Bayes' theorem. *N Engl J Med*. **293**: 257.

Clinical Bottom Line

A child who feels normal or cool to their mother or medical personnel, is very unlikely to have a temperature. This finding can be clinically useful in ruling out the presence of a temperature (SnNout).

Citation

Whybrew K, Murray M, Morley C (1998) Diagnosing fever by touch: observational study. *BMJ.* **317:** 321.

Clinical Question

In a child in whom fever is suspected, can feeling warm to the touch be used to diagnose fever, and can feeling normal or cool to the touch be used to exclude fever?

Search Terms

'temperature' and ('sensitivity and specificity')

The Study

1   Gold standard – axillary temperature measured by thermometer.

2   Study setting – patients aged one month to 16 years attending a Zambian hospital.

The subjects were examined by a medical student and their mother, who formed a judgement on whether they felt warm/hot or normal/cold.

The Evidence

	Temperature >37.8	Temperature <37.8	Likelihood ratio
Mother feels:			
Child warm or hot	221	353	1.7
Child normal or cold	15	273	0.14
Students feel:			
Child warm or hot	257	268	2.8
Child normal or cold	17	544	0.09

Comments

1   Not clear how the patient sample was assembled.

2   Feeling normal or cool to the touch is a SnNout for temperature.

EBM SESSION

3

Prognosis
and
searching the
evidence-
based
journals

PART A | Critical appraisal of a clinical article about prognosis

You see a 70-year old man on outpatient follow-up, three months after his discharge from your hospital with an ischaemic (presumed thrombotic) stroke. He is in sinus rhythm, has mild residual left-sided weakness, but is otherwise well. He had an upper gastrointestinal bleed while on aspirin a few years earlier, so he is on no medications. His sister-in-law scared him last week by telling him he will probably die by the year's end, and he wants to know what the chance is that this will happen to him.

You form the question: 'In a 70-year old man who has had a thrombotic stroke, what is the risk of death within the first year?'

You search *Best Evidence* by typing in 'stroke prognosis' and find 'Mortality in first-ever stroke'. Although it gives you a quick answer (in the form of a structured abstract and clinical commentary) in a few seconds, you decide to read the original paper: *Stroke* (1993) **24:** 796–800).

Read the article and decide:
1 Is this evidence about prognosis valid?
2 Is this valid evidence about prognosis important?
3 Can you apply this valid and important evidence about prognosis in caring for your patient?

If you want to read some strategies for answering these sorts of questions, you could have a look at pp 85–90, 129–32 and 164–5 in *Evidence-based Medicine*.

PART B | Searching the evidence-based journals

We show you how to search the electronic version of two journals: *ACP Journal Club (ACPJC)* and *Evidence-based Medicine*. The contents of these journals are available on disk as *Best Evidence*. This requires a computer with a CD slot and can be ordered from the BMJ Publishing Group, PO Box 295, London WC1H 9TE; Tel: 0171 387 4499 (subscriptions); Fax: 0171 383 6662; e-mail: bmjsubs@dial.pipex.com.

You might try out searching these evidence-based journals for answers to some of the questions you generated last week.

Now would be a good time to start searching on potential topics for your presentations in Sessions 6 and 7!

Long-term Survival After First-Ever Stroke: The Oxfordshire Community Stroke Project

Martin S. Dennis, MD; John P.S. Burn, DM; Peter A.G. Sandercock, DM; John M. Bamford, MD; Derick T. Wade, MD; and Charles P. Warlow, MD

Background and Purpose: There have been relatively few community-based studies of long-term prognosis after acute stroke. This study aimed to provide precise estimates of the absolute and relative risks of dying in an unselected cohort of patients with a first-ever stroke.

Methods: Six hundred seventy-five patients were registered by a community-based stroke register (the Oxfordshire Community Stroke Project) and prospectively followed up for up to 6.5 years. Their relative risk of death was calculated using age- and sex-specific mortality rates for Oxfordshire.

Results: During the first 30 days, 129 (19%) patients died. Patients who survived at least 30 days after a first-ever stroke thereafter had an average annual risk of death of 9.1%, 2.3-fold the risk in people from the general population. Although the absolute (about 15%) and relative (about threefold) risks of death were highest in these 30-day survivors over the first year after the stroke, they were at increased risk of dying over the next few years (range of relative risk for individual years, 1.1–2.9). Predictably, older patients had a worse absolute survival but, relative to the general population, stroke also increased the relative risk of dying in younger patients. During the first 30 days stroke accounts for most deaths; after this time nonstroke cardiovascular disease becomes increasingly important and is the most common cause of death after the first year.

Conclusions: These data highlight the importance of long-term secondary prevention of vascular events in stroke patients, targeted as much at the cardiovascular as at the cerebrovascular circulation. (*Stroke* 1993;24:796–800)

KEY WORDS • epidemiology • Great Britain • prognosis • survival

The risk of death from stroke is highest in the first few weeks after the stroke, although reported 30-day case fatality rates vary widely. Hospital-based studies may report higher early case fatality rates than community-based studies because they include a larger proportion of patients with severe or recurrent strokes, sometimes associated with other nonstroke illnesses. In the Oxfordshire Community Stroke Project (OCSP) the 30-day case fatality rate after a first-ever in a lifetime stroke (first stroke) was 19%.[1] Most of the deaths in the first week resulted from direct damage to the brain, whereas deaths in the subsequent few weeks resulted from complications of immobility (e.g., pneumonia, pulmonary embolism) and less frequently from further vascular events such as recurrent stroke or myocardial infarction.[2] There have been relatively few studies of long-term survival, and even fewer that have

been community based[3–7] and therefore able to report the long-term prognosis of an unselected cohort. In hospital-referred cohorts, the absolute risk of death may be higher and less readily generalizable because referral patterns vary from one hospital to another, and such series are likely to include an unknown and variable excess of patients with severe and recurrent strokes and other illnesses. Alternatively, one might argue that the high early case fatality rate in hospital-referred series may select patients with a good long-term prognosis (i.e., survival effect). Long-term data on the risk of death from all causes, and more specifically deaths from vascular causes, are needed in clinical practice, in the design of clinical trials, and in the planning of health care delivery. In this article we describe the long-term absolute and relative risks of death in an unselected sample of patients with a first stroke in the OCSP.

Methods

Six hundred seventy-five patients with a first stroke were identified prospectively by the OCSP and followed up to establish their long-term prognosis. The study population, clinical definitions, methods employed to ensure complete case ascertainment, methods of assessment, and investigations have been described in detail elsewhere.[8] Surviving patients were followed up by one of two trained research nurses at 1, 6, and 12 months and then annually from the date of stroke onset. At each follow-up visit, the patient was questioned carefully about any symptoms of transient ischemic attack, recur-

From the Department of Clinical Neurosciences (M.S.D., P.A.G.S., C.P.W.), Western General Hospital, Edinburgh; the Department of Rehabilitation Medicine (J.P.S.B.), Southampton General Hospital, Southampton; the Department of Neurology (J.M.B.), St. James's University Hospital, Leeds; and the Rivermead Rehabilitation Centre (D.T.W.), Oxford, U.K.

Supported by the Medical Research Council of Great Britain and the Stroke Association.

Address for correspondence: Dr. Martin S. Dennis, Department of Clinical Neurosciences, Western General Hospital, Edinburgh, U.K., EH4 2XU.

Received December 1, 1992; final revision received January 18, 1993; accepted February 17, 1993.

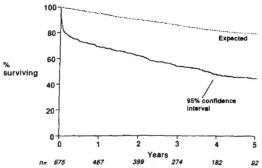

FIGURE 1. *Kaplan-Meier survival curves showing the probability of survival after a first-ever stroke. The shading indicates 95% confidence intervals. The expected survival was calculated from the mortality rates for Oxfordshire, England.*[14]

rent stroke, and myocardial infarction; if the nurse suspected that one of these might have occurred, the patient was reassessed by a study neurologist. During 1988 all surviving patients were seen for a more detailed assessment by one of us (J.P.S.B.). When a patient died we reviewed all available hospital, general practitioner, and autopsy records. The cause of death was determined by using all the available clinical evidence rather than just the death certificate, which may be inaccurate.[9,10] For the purposes of this article we classified deaths into five groups: 1) First stroke deaths were due to the direct effects of the brain lesion or due to complications of immobility resulting from the first stroke. These included deaths from bronchopneumonia even several years after the stroke, if stroke-related impairments were thought to be in some way responsible and there was no other, more likely, cause of death. 2) Recurrent stroke deaths were directly due to the brain lesion or complications of immobility following a severe recurrent stroke (i.e., with symptoms that lasted a week or led to early death and were associated with an increase in disability). If deaths from stroke-related impairments occurred after a severe recurrent stroke they were viewed as being due to the recurrent stroke

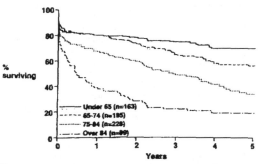

FIGURE 2. *Kaplan-Meier survival curves showing the probability of survival in patients with a first-ever stroke stratified by age. There was a significant trend (χ^2 trend, 75.8; p<0.001) for older patients to have a worse survival.*

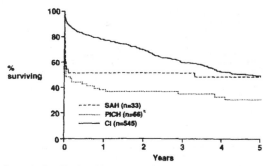

FIGURE 3. *Kaplan-Meier survival curves showing the probability of survival in patients with a first-ever stroke due to cerebral infarction (CI), primary intracerebral hemorrhage (PICH), and subarachnoid hemorrhage (SAH).*

rather than the first stroke. 3) Cardiovascular deaths were those due to definite or probable cardiac causes, ruptured aortic aneurysm, or peripheral vascular disease. Sudden deaths were regarded as cardiovascular unless an alternative explanation was found at autopsy. 4) Nonvascular deaths were unrelated to any stroke disability and clearly due to a nonvascular cause, e.g., cancer, accidents, or suicide. 5) Unclassified deaths were those in which there was so little information that no cause could be given.

We have described survival using actuarial analysis, in which day 0 was taken as the date of first stroke. Kaplan-Meier survival curves are given with 95% confidence intervals[11] (CIs). The average annual risk of death was calculated by using the method described by Hankey et al.[12] The risk of death for the stroke patients was compared with that for people of similar age and sex from the same general population who were assumed to be stroke free; this was calculated by using the person-years program[13] using age- and sex-specific mortality statistics for Oxfordshire.[14] Approximate 95% CIs of relative risks were calculated using the Poisson distribution.

Results

Six hundred seventy-five patients with a first stroke were identified in the study population during a 4-year

TABLE 1. **Relative Risk of Dying After a First-Ever Stroke During Different Time Intervals From Stroke Onset for Patients of All Ages**

Intervals	Number at risk	Observed deaths	Expected deaths	O/E	95% Confidence interval
Year 1	675	208	28.0	7.4	6.5–8.5
Year 2	467	46	24.5	1.9	1.4–2.5
Year 3	399	45	18.0	2.5	1.8–3.4
Year 4	274	31	14.3	2.2	1.5–3.1
Year 5	182	8	7.1	1.1	0.5–2.2
Year 6	92	9	3.2	2.9	1.3–5.4
30 days–6 years	546	218	93.1	2.3	2.0–2.7
All intervals	675	347	95.0	3.7	3.3–4.1

O/E, observed deaths/expected deaths.

TABLE 2.   **Relative Risk of Dying After a First-Ever Stroke in Patients of Different Ages for All Time Intervals**

Age	Number at risk	Observed deaths	Expected deaths	O/E	95% Confidence interval
<45 years	26	3	0.1	37.5	6.2–87.7
45–54 years	25	8	0.3	25.8	11.1–50.8
55–64 years	112	32	3.0	10.6	7.3–14.9
65–74 years	195	75	15.6	4.8	3.8–6.0
75–84 years	228	145	44.3	3.3	2.8–3.9
>84 years	89	84	31.8	2.7	2.1–3.3
All ages	675	347	95.0	3.7	3.3–4.1

O/E, observed deaths/expected deaths.

period. Their mean age was 72 years; 318 (47%) were male. The pathological type of the first stroke was cerebral infarction in 545 (81%), primary intracerebral hemorrhage in 66 (10%), subarachnoid hemorrhage in 33 (5%), and unknown pathological type in 31 (5%). Surviving patients were followed up for a minimum of 2 years and up to 6.5 years. By the end of the follow-up period, 347 (51%) patients had died. An autopsy was conducted in 56 (43%) of the 129 patients dying in the first 30 days, but in only 44 (20%) of the 218 dying thereafter. No patient was lost to follow-up.

Absolute Risks for All Patients

A Kaplan-Meier survival curve for all 675 patients is shown in Figure 1. The risks of death over the first 30 days and over the first year were about 19% (95% CI, 16–22%) and 31% (95% CI, 27–34%), respectively. For those surviving at least 30 days or for at least 1 year, the average annual risks of death up to 5 years were 9.1% (95% CI, 8.1–10.4%) and 6.6% (95% CI, 4.6–8.8%), respectively. In 30-day survivors the risk of dying was higher in the remainder of the first year (about 15%) than in subsequent years.

Absolute Risks for Subgroups

Stratification by age showed that older patients had a worse prognosis (χ^2 trend, 75.8; $p<0.001$), both during the early period after the stroke and throughout the follow-up period (Figure 2). There was a nonsignificant trend for women to have a worse prognosis than men, but this disappeared after correcting for differences in age (age-adjusted relative odds, M:F=0.93; 95% CI, 0.74–1.15%). The survival curves comparing prognosis in the different pathological types of stroke are shown in Figure 3. As we have demonstrated previously,[1] the

survival curves diverge over the first 30 days but, because few ($n=50$) patients with intracranial hemorrhage survived beyond 30 days, comparisons of late survival are unreliable, although the long-term risk of death after primary intracerebral hemorrhage did seem similar to the risk after cerebral infarction. The risk of dying in the first year after a first stroke due to cerebral infarction was 22.1% (95% CI, 18.9–26.9%). In cerebral infarction patients who were alive at the end of the first year, the average annual risk of death over the next 4 years was 8.5% (95% CI, 6.1–10.5%). The long-term prognosis for 30-day survivors of subarachnoid hemorrhage was good, with only two of 18 survivors dying subsequently, which may reflect their relatively young age and the protective effect of aneurysm surgery.

Relative Risk Compared With General Population

The risk of dying after a first stroke compared with the risk of death in people of similar age and sex in the general population is shown in Tables 1 and 2. The relative risk is given for each yearly interval from the onset of stroke (Table 1) and for different age bands (Table 2). In the first year stroke patients had a 7.4-fold risk (95% CI, 6.5–8.5%) of death varying between 1.1 and 2.9 in subsequent years. Patients who survived at least 30 days had approximately a threefold greater risk of dying in the next year than people in the general population. The relative risk was far greater in younger patients. In the first year the relative risk of dying in a 45–54-year-old was 71.8 (95% CI, 27.5–163.3%) compared with a relative risk for all ages in the first year of 7.4 (95% CI, 6.5–8.5%). In the second and third years, the relative risk of dying in younger patients remained higher, though this was based on very few deaths (two in the 45–54-year-old age group), so that we cannot be certain whether younger survivors of stroke have continuing increased risk of dying compared with stroke-free individuals. The relative risk for all stroke patients of all ages was 3.7 over the first 6 years, and for those surviving 30 days the subsequent relative risk was 2.3 (95% CI, 2.0–2.7%). For all ages combined, the relative risk of death over the first year after cerebral infarction (all ages) was 4.8 (95% CI, 4.2–5.7%) and 2.1 (95% CI, 1.8–2.5%) over the next 5 years.

Causes of Death

Table 3 and Figure 4 show the causes of death during different time intervals from the onset of the first stroke. For those patients who survived at least 30 days, 36% of subsequent deaths were due to the first or recurrent

TABLE 3.   **Causes of Death Within Different Time Intervals After a First-Ever Stroke**

Causes of death	Number of deaths within each time interval								
	0–30 days *n*	30 Days–6 months *n*	6 Months–1 year *n*	1–2 Years *n*	2–3 Years *n*	3–4 Years *n*	4–5 Years *n*	5–6 Years *n*	All intervals
First stroke	116 (90)	22 (44)	8 (28)	5 (11)	3 (7)	1 (3)	0 (0)	2 (22)	157
Recurrent stroke	1 (1)	9 (18)	6 (21)	7 (15)	5 (11)	8 (26)	0 (0)	2 (22)	38
Nonstroke/ cardiovascular	9 (7)	11 (22)	9 (31)	24 (56)	10 (22)	14 (45)	3 (38)	4 (44)	84
Nonvascular	3 (2)	8 (16)	5 (17)	9 (20)	26 (58)	8 (26)	4 (50)	1 (11)	64
Unknown	0 (0)	0 (0)	1 (3)	1 (2)	1 (2)	0 (0)	1 (12)	0 (0)	4
All causes	129	50	29	46	45	31	8	9	347

Numbers in parentheses are percent of deaths.

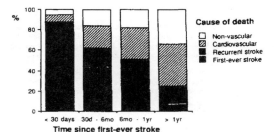

FIGURE 4. *Histogram showing the proportion of patients dying from different causes during different time intervals from the onset of their first-ever stroke.*

stroke, whereas 34% were due to other vascular causes. Of the patients who survived at least 30 days after their first stroke due to cerebral infarction but who then died during the follow-up period, 33 (17%) died of their first stroke, 32 (16%) died as a result of recurrent stroke, 70 (35%) died of a nonstroke cardiovascular cause, and 60 (30%) died of nonvascular causes. In four (2%) the cause of death was unknown. Among the patients with primary intracerebral hemorrhage, subarachnoid hemorrhage, and unknown pathology, there were only 19 deaths after 30 days, so that no conclusions could be drawn from these data.

Conclusions

This study is important because it is community-based and therefore provides an unselected series of first-stroke patients for study; there was a prospective neurological assessment; a large proportion of stroke patients underwent a CT scan or autopsy to determine the pathological type of stroke; follow-up was prospective and prolonged; and it provides estimates of relative as well as absolute risks. Table 4 shows the only other studies that were community based and have published long-term (at least 5-year) survival data.

The risk of dying over the first 5 years after stroke is similar in the different studies and is probably not statistically significantly different except for that from Moscow,[3] where 72% (95% CI, 70–74%) of the study subjects died compared with risks of 45% (95% CI, 37.7–51.5%)[4] to 61% (95% CI, 51.4–70.6%)[6] in the other studies. (Scmidt et al[3] gave the actual rather than the actuarial risk, although this was comparable because all patients appear to have been followed up for at least 5 years or until death.) This poorer survival may have been, in part, because the Moscow study[3] included recurrent strokes in their inception cohort. The study with the next worse prognosis[6] may also have included recurrent strokes in their inception cohort. Perhaps of more interest is the relative risk of dying in stroke patients compared with people in the general population in the different studies. Our study suggests that patients have a persistent and statistically significant excess risk of death for several years after their first stroke. Sacco et al,[4] using data from the Framingham study, also demonstrated that the excess risk of dying persists for several years, although those without coexistent hypertension or heart disease had no excess risk if they survived the first year. This suggested to the authors that any excess risk of death was related to such coexistent problems rather than to the stroke itself. Data from Rochester, Minnesota[15] suggested that patients who had survived at least a year after a stroke had little or no excess risk of death in subsequent years; there may have been several methodological reasons for this difference, but the most likely is simply the small number of patients and the very small number of deaths, which gave imprecise estimates of relative risk. Failure to show a significant excess of deaths after year 1 may have been a false-negative (type 2) error. Indeed, these previous studies have not provided any measure of the precision of their results. Even in our study the estimates of excess risk were fairly imprecise (see 95% CIs in Tables 1 and 2).

TABLE 4. **Comparison of Risk of Death After Stroke in Community-Based Studies**

Study	Diagnosis	Actuarial risk of death (%)		
		30 Days	By 1 year	By 5 years
OCSP	Cerebral infarction	10	23	52
	PICH	52	62	70
	SAH	45	48	52
	All first-ever strokes	19	31	45
Framingham[4]	Cerebral infarction	15	NA	NA
	PICH	82	NA	NA
	SAH	46	NA	NA
	All first-ever strokes	22	NA	Men 48
				Women 40
Rochester[15]	Cerebral infarction	16	NA	52
	PICH	58	NA	NA
	SAH	37	NA	NA
	All first-ever strokes	23	39	54
Moscow[3]	All strokes	37	52	72
Ikawa[6]	All strokes	NA	32	61

OCSP, Oxfordshire Community Stroke Project; PICH, primary intracerebral hemorrhage; SAH, subarachnoid hemorrhage; NA, not available.

800   **Stroke** *Vol 24, No 6 June 1993*

Our data confirm that the risk of death early after a first stroke is high, which supports the worldwide efforts to identify medical treatments to improve early prognosis. Although deaths due to stroke are proportionally the most important early on, in subsequent years deaths due to recurrent stroke and in particular those due to cardiovascular problems become numerically more important. The finding that stroke patients have a significant excess risk of death even after the first year demonstrates a clear need for prolonged secondary prevention aimed equally at the heart and cerebral circulations.

Acknowledgments

We wish to thank all those who have helped with this project, including Sue Price, Liz Mogridge, and Claire Clifford, our study nurses; Lesley Jones, the project computer programmer; and Helen Storrie, Venessa Langsbury, Angie Dwyer, and Andrea Watts, who provided secretarial support. We especially thank our collaborating general practitioners, without whom this project would be impossible. The collaborating practices were (name of liaison partner from each practice only): Dr. A. MacPherson, Oxford; Dr. A. Marcus, Thames; Dr. D. Leggate, Oxford; Dr. M. Agass, Berinsfield; Dr. D. Otterburn, Abingdon; Dr. S. Street, Kidlington; Dr. V. Drury, Wantage; Dr. R. Pinches, Abingdon; Dr. N. Crossley, Abingdon; and Dr. H. O'Donnell, Deddington.

References

1. Bamford J, Sandercock P, Dennis M, Burn J, Warlow C: A prospective study of acute cerebrovascular disease in the community: The Oxfordshire Community Stroke Project—1981–1986: 2. Incidence, case fatality rates and overall outcome at one year of cerebral infarction, primary intracerebral and subarachnoid haemorrhage. *J Neurol Neurosurg Psychiatry* 1990;53:16–22
2. Bamford J, Dennis M, Sandercock P, Burn J, Warlow C: The frequency, causes and timing of death within 30 days of a first stroke: The Oxfordshire Community Stroke Project. *J Neurol Neurosurg Psychiatry* 1990;53:824–829
3. Scmidt EV, Smirnov VE, Ryabova VS: Results of the seven-year prospective study of stroke patients. *Stroke* 1988;19:942–949
4. Sacco RL, Wolf PA, Kannel WB, McNamara PM: Survival and recurrence following stroke: The Framingham study. *Stroke* 1982; 13:290–296
5. Matsumoto N, Whisnant JP, Kurland LT, Okazaki H: Natural history of stroke in Rochester, Minnesota, 1955 through 1969: An extension of a previous study, 1945 through 1954. *Stroke* 1973;4: 20–29
6. Kojima S, Omura T, Wakamatsu W, Kishi M, Yamazaki T, Iida M, Komachi Y: Prognosis and disability of stroke patients after 5 Years in Akita, Japan. *Stroke* 1990;21:72–77
7. Garraway WM, Whisnant JP, Drury I: The changing pattern of survival following stroke. *Stroke* 1983;14:699–703
8. Bamford J, Sandercock P, Dennis M, Warlow C, Jones L, MacPherson K, Vessey M, Fowler G, Molyneux A, Hughes T, Burn J, Wade D: A prospective study of acute cerebrovascular disease in the community: The Oxfordshire Community Stroke Project—1981–1986: 1. Methodology, demography and incidence cases of first-ever stroke. *J Neurol Neurosurg Psychiatry* 1988;51: 1373–1380
9. Cameron HM, McGoogan E: A prospective study of 1152 hospital autopsies: 1. Inaccuracies in death certification. *J Pathol* 1981;133: 273–283
10. Cameron HM, McGoogan E: A prospective study of 1152 hospital autopsies: 2. Analysis of inaccuracies in clinical diagnosis and their significance. *J Pathol* 1981;133:285–300
11. Machin D, Gardner MJ: Calculating confidence intervals for survival time analyses, in Gardner MJ, Altman DG (eds): *Statistics With Confidence.* Belfast, Br Med J, 1989, pp 64–70
12. Hankey GJ, Slattery JM, Warlow CP: The prognosis of hospital referred transient ischaemic attacks. *J Neurol Neurosurg Psychiatry* 1991;54:793–802
13. Coleman M, Douglas A, Herman C, Peto J: Cohort study analysis with a fortran computer program. *Int J Epidemiol* 1986;15:134–137
14. Office of Population, Census and Surveys: *Mortality Statistics 1985.* London, Her Majesty's Stationery Office, 1987
15. Dyken ML: Natural history of ischaemic stroke in cerebrovascular disease, in Harrison MJG, Dyken ML (eds): *Butterworth International Medical Reviews: Neurology,* ed 3. London, Butterworth, 1983, pp 139–170

Citation:

Are the results of this prognosis study valid?

Was a defined, representative sample of patients assembled at a common (usually early) point in the course of their disease?

Was patient follow-up sufficiently long and complete?

Were objective outcome criteria applied in a 'blind' fashion?

If subgroups with different prognoses are identified, was there adjustment for important prognostic factors?

Was there validation in an independent group ('test-set') of patients?

Are the valid results of this prognosis study important?

How likely are the outcomes over time?

How precise are the prognostic estimates?

If you want to calculate a confidence interval around the measure of prognosis

(*see* Appendix 1 in *Evidence-based Medicine*)

Clinical Measure	Standard Error (SE)	Typical calculation of CI
Proportion (as in the rate of some prognostic event, etc.) where: the number of patients = n the proportion of these patients who experience the event = p	$\sqrt{\{p \times (1-p)/n\}}$ where p is proportion and n is number of patients	If p = 24/60 = 0.4 (or 40%) and n = 60 $SE = \sqrt{\{0.4 \times (1-0.4)/60\}}$ = 0.063 (or 6.3%) 95% CI is 40% +/− 1.96 x 6.3% or 27.6% to 52.4%
n from your evidence: _____ p from your evidence: _____	$\sqrt{\{p \times (1-p)/n\}}$ where p is proportion and n is number of patients	Your calculation: SE: _____ 95% CI: _____

Can you apply this valid, important evidence about prognosis in caring for your patient?

Were the study patients similar to your own?

Will this evidence make a clinically important impact on your conclusions about what to offer or tell your patient?

Additional notes

Citation: Dennis MS, Burn JP, Sandercock PA *et al.* (1993) Long-term survival after first-ever stroke: The Oxfordshire Community Stroke Project. *Stroke.* 24: 796–800.

Are the results of this prognosis study valid?

Was a defined, representative sample of patients assembled at a common (usually early) point in the course of their disease?	**Yes. From a common starting point but we don't know how GP's decided which stroke patients to send to hospital.**
Was patient follow-up sufficiently long and complete?	**Yes. For a minimum of 2 years and up to 6.5 years.**
Were objective outcome criteria applied in a 'blind' fashion?	**Objective outcome criteria were applied but observations were not blinded.**
If subgroups with different prognoses are identified, was there adjustment for important prognostic factors?	**Some stratification by age and type of stroke, but not for clinically relevant subgroups (these are reported in a later paper: *Stroke* (1994) 25: 333–37).**
Was there validation in an independent group ('test-set') of patients?	**No.**

Are the valid results of this prognosis study important?

How likely are the outcomes over time?	**The estimate for our patient dying in the first year after a cerebral infarction was 22%, but because he's already survived the first month's high risk, his chance of dying in the remainder of the first year are less than half that.**
How precise are the prognostic estimates?	**The 95% confidence interval on that 22% runs from 19% to 27%, so it's pretty precise.**

If you want to calculate a confidence interval around the measure of prognosis

(*see* Appendix 1 in *Evidence-based Medicine*)

Clinical Measure	Standard Error (SE)	Typical calculation of CI
Proportion (as in the rate of some prognostic event, etc.) where: the number of patients = n the proportion of these patients who experience the event = p	$\sqrt{\{p \times (1-p)/n\}}$ where p is proportion and n is number of patients	If p = 24/60 = 0.4 (or 40%) and n = 60 $SE = \sqrt{\{0.4 \times (1-0.4)/60\}}$ = 0.063 (or 6.3%) 95% CI is 40% +/− 1.96 x 6.3% or 27.6% to 52.4%
n from your evidence: **675** p from your evidence: **0.22**	$\sqrt{\{p \times (1-p)/n\}}$ where p is proportion and n is number of patients	Your calculation: SE: **0.016** 95% CI: **+/− 3%**

Can you apply this valid, important evidence about prognosis in caring for your patient?

Were the study patients similar to your own?	**Yes.**
Will this evidence make a clinically important impact on your conclusions about what to offer or tell your patient?	**In this patient, yes.**

Additional notes

For clinical subgroups, see *Stroke* (1994) 25: 333–37.

ACP Journal Club (1993) Nov–Dec: **119**: 83.

Based on: Dennis MS, Burn JP, Sandercock PA *et al.* (1993) Long-term survival after first-ever stroke: The Oxfordshire Community Stroke Project. *Stroke.* **24**: 796–800.

Objective

To determine the incidence of death after a first-ever stroke in patients registered with the Oxfordshire Community Stroke Project.

Design

Inception cohort followed for a maximum of 6.5 years.

Setting

Population-based study in the United Kingdom.

Patients

675 patients (mean age, 72 years; 53% women) with a first stroke identified in a community-based stroke register. The pathologic type of the first stroke was cerebral infarction in 545 (81%), primary intracerebral hemorrhage in 66 (10%), subarachnoid hemorrhage in 33 (5%), and unknown in 31 (5%).

Assessment of prognostic factors

Age, gender and pathologic type of the first stroke were noted. Follow-up assessments were done at one, six, and 12 months, and annually thereafter. Symptoms of transient ischemic attack, recurrent stroke and myocardial infarction were documented.

Main outcome measures

Mortality classified as first-stroke deaths, recurrent-stroke deaths, cardiovascular deaths, non-vascular deaths, and unclassified deaths. The cause of death was determined by reviewing all available clinical evidence including hospital, general practitioner and autopsy records.

Main results

The risks for death during the first 30 days and during the first year were 19% (CI, 16% to 22%) and 31% (CI, 27% to 34%), respectively. For those surviving at least 30 days or for at least one year, the average annual risks for death up to five years were 9.1% (CI, 8.1% to 10.4%) and 6.6% (CI, 4.6% to 8.8%), respectively. In patients who survived for 30 days, the risk for dying during the rest of the first year was 15% higher than in subsequent years. Stratification by age showed that older patients had a worse prognosis during the early period after the stroke and throughout the follow-up period (P < 0.001). The risk for dying in the first year after a first stroke caused by cerebral infarction was 22.1% (CI, 18.9% to 26.9%). The data on the risks for dying in the first year because of intracranial hemorrhage and subarachnoid hemorrhage were unreliable because few patients survived beyond 30 days. For those patients who survived at least 30 days, 36% of deaths were caused by the first or recurrent stroke, and 34% were because of other vascular causes.

Conclusions

In an unselected, community-based population with first stroke, the risk for dying remained elevated for several years but was particularly high in the first 30 days.

Sources of funding: Medical Research Council of Great Britain and the Stroke Association.

For article reprint: Dr MS Dennis, Department of Clinical Neurosciences, Western General Hospital, Edinburgh, United Kingdom EH4 2XU. Fax: 0131 332 5150.

ACP Journal Club Commentary

The study by Dennis and colleagues is important because it is community-based. Patients presenting with stroke are very high-risk patients who should be treated aggressively, not only with medical treatment for atherosclerotic risk factors, such as hyperlipidemia.[1] They should also be considered for carotid endarterectomy in appropriate circumstances. The North American Symptomatic Carotid Endarterectomy Trial (NASCET) showed a reduction in 2-year risk for stroke and death from 24% in the group randomised to medical therapy (a risk figure remarkably close to that reported in the study by Dennis and colleagues) to 9% in patients randomised to surgery for symptomatic severe (70%) carotid stenosis.[2] The high risk reported in the study by Dennis and colleagues supports the observation that it is no longer adequate management for patients with stroke or transient ischemic attacks to simply recommend that they take aspirin and cross their fingers. The cause of the stroke must be identified; if they have severe symptomatic carotid stenosis and are medically fit for surgery and an expert surgeon is available, endarterectomy should be offered.

In this study, intracerebral hemorrhage accounted for only 10% of first strokes. Improved detection and treatment of hypertension may have led to a decline in the proportion of strokes caused by intracerebral hemorrhage.[3]

J David Spence, MD
University of Western Ontario
London, Ontario.

References

1 Bots ML, Breslau PJ, Briet E *et al.* (1992) Cardiovascular determinants of carotid artery disease. The Rotterdam elderly study. *Hypertension.* **19:** 717–20.
2 North American Symptomatic Carotid Endarterectomy Trial Collaborators (1991) Beneficial effect of carotid endarterectomy in symptomatic patients with high-grade carotid stenosis. *NEJM.* **325:** 445–53.
3 Spence JD (1986) Antihypertensive drugs and prevention of atherosclerotic stroke. *Stroke.* **17:** 808–10.

STROKE – PROGNOSIS AT ONE YEAR

Appraised by Sharon Straus,
October 1996.
Expiry date: 1998.

Clinical Bottom Line

A patient with an ischaemic stroke, who is not on any antiplatelet agents or anticoagulants and is otherwise well, has a 22% risk of dying within the first year.

Citation

Denis MS, Burn JP, Sandercock PA *et al.* (1993) Long-term survival after first-ever stroke: The Oxfordshire Community Stroke Project. *Stroke.* **24:** 796–800.

Clinical Question

In a patient with thrombotic stroke, what is the risk of death within the first year?

Search Terms

'stroke prognosis' in *Best Evidence.*

The Study

Cohort of 675 patients registered in a community-based stroke registry followed up prospectively for up to 6.5 years.

The Evidence

Group	Event	Timing	Rate	95% CI
Ischaemic strokes	Death	One year	22%	19% to 27%
All strokes	Death	One month	19%	16% to 22%
All strokes	Death	One year	31%	27% to 34%
All strokes who survived first year	Death	Annual death rate for years 2–5	6.6%	4.6% to 8.8%

Comments

1 Unsure how physicians selected patients for registration.

2 Not all potentially important prognostic factors adjusted for, e.g. antiplatelet therapy, use of anticoagulants, a fib and size of the left atrium.

3 Outcome observers were not blinded.

4 Some outcome events were not picked up until the next follow-up visit, which could have been up to a year after the event – investigators had to rely on patient information and medical records in that case.

5 For subgroups, see later paper: *Stroke* (1994) **25:** 333–7.

SOURCES OF EVIDENCE FOR EVIDENCE-BASED MEDICINE

Title	Medium	Content type	Advantages	Disadvantages
Best Evidence on Disk (American College of Physicians & BMJ Publications Group)	CD-ROM or diskette (cumulated contents of two paper journals: *ACP Journal Club* and *Evidence-based Medicine.*) Updated every year.	Structured abstracts of articles from selected journals in internal medicine, general practice, obstetrics and gynaecology, paediatrics, psychiatry, and surgery. Articles must meet strict quality criteria; each abstract (evidence) accompanied by a commentary (clinical expertise).	High quality evidence with commentary; easy to search; high specificity (not much time wasted with irrelevant material).	Incomplete coverage of literature: low sensitivity.

WHEN TO USE IT: *As your first port of call for the specialities it covers.*

Cochrane Library	CD-ROM or diskette or Internet	Superb evidence about therapy & prevention; thousands of world-wide systematic reviews; abstracts of overviews of effectiveness.	Highest quality evidence we'll ever have on the effectiveness of health care.	Not yet many Cochrane reviews; necessarily omits the newest treatments.

WHEN TO USE IT: *As your best port of call for therapy.*

MEDLINE (US National Library of Medicine)	Networked CD-ROM systems; on-line vendors. (SilverPlatter [WinSPIRS] Ovid, etc.)	Bibliographic records, with abstract and MeSH terms. Full-text services starting to appear.	Exhaustiveness; flexibility of searching; journal coverage; currency (on-line versions); widespread availability and support (lots of people can help you!)	Have to do your own quality filtering; putting together good searches is difficult; gaps in coverage (medical, geographical and linguistic).

WHEN TO USE IT: *When you need to be sure you've got everything and have time to search properly.*

World-Wide Web (WWW)	Internet (via browser programs such as Netscape, MS Internet Explorer, Mosaic, Yahoo, Lynx, etc.)	Everything: from LRs to NNTs; electronic journals (e.g. Bandolier) & journal clubs; software tools; CATs; teaching materials; searching tips; events and conferences; etc.	Some sites are excellent, with high-quality pre-filtered evidence; some good, free software; boundless possibilities; can be updated instantly.	Variable levels of quality control; poor sensitivity and specificity; access from NHS networks can be problematic; can be slow to download.

WHEN TO USE IT: *Find good sites and check them regularly for updates.*

Recommended sites:	CEBM	http://cebm.jr2.ox.ac.uk/	CATs, NNTs, LRs, etc., teaching materials, announcements, links to other sites.	
	SCHARR / AurACLE	http://www.shef.ac.uk/~scharr/ir/netting.html	Evidence-based information seeking, links to other sites.	
	Bandolier	http://www.jr2.ox.ac.uk/Bandolier/	An electronic version (including back issues) of the EBM journal *Bandolier.*	
WWW search services	General comment on Web searching	Allow you to type in keywords and search an index of WWW pages.	Tens of millions of pages are indexed and can be accessed directly. Searching is crude and hits displayed in an order which is not always appropriate.	
Typical specific services:	Yahoo!	http://www.yahoo.com	More selective than most search sites, though this may not coincide with your needs!	
	AltaVista	http://www.altavista.com	Seems to be the most exhaustive, with best searching engine.	

WHEN TO USE IT: *To find very specific information from the Web or starting points for browsing.*

PART A Critical appraisal of a clinical article about harm

A 49-year old woman attends your surgery. Her periods have recently stopped and she has developed hot flushes and vaginal dryness, symptoms which she recognizes to be typical of the menopause. She has come to discuss the pros and cons of hormone replacement therapy (HRT). She is a non-smoker and has a normal blood pressure. She took the oral contraceptive pill from the age of 25–35. Age 35, she broke her leg in a bicycle accident. While recovering from this, and while still taking the oral contraceptive pill, she suffered a deep vein thrombosis (proven by venogram). Haematological testing did not identify a known thrombophilic factor in her blood, but she was advised to use another method of contraception. She wants to know if HRT puts her at risk of deep vein thrombosis (DVT).

You form the clinical question: 'In post-menopausal women does hormone replacement therapy lead to an increased risk of deep vein thrombosis, and if so, what is the size of the risk?'

A MEDLINE search using the MeSH term 'thromboembolism', the text word 'HRT' and the text word 'risk' for MEDLINE 1996–8 yielded nine studies, of which two (both published in the same issue of the *Lancet*) looked like they addressed our question. We scrutinised both abstracts, and then asked the library to fax a copy of: Daly E, Vessey MP, Hawkins MM *et al.* (1996) Risk of venous thromboembolism in users of hormone replacement therapy. *Lancet.* **348**(9033): 977–80.

Read this article and decide:
1 Are the results of this harm study valid?
2 Are the results of this harm study important?
3 Should these valid, important results of this study about a potentially harmful treatment change the treatment of your patient?

If you want to read some strategies for answering these sorts of questions, you could have a look at pp 105–10, 147–9 and 179–81 in *Evidence-based Medicine*.

PART B Searching for evidence in the primary literature

Colleagues from the library will whet your appetite for learning how to search for evidence in the clinical literature (or hone the searching skills you already have developed), so bring along the clinical questions you generated in Session 2 (or any that you have generated in the meantime). Efficient EBM searching strategies (that trade off the sensitivity and specificity of your searches) are included.

BEST SINGLE TERMS AND COMBINATIONS FOR HIGH SENSITIVITY MEDLINE SEARCHES ON THE BEST STUDIES OF TREATMENT, DIAGNOSIS, PROGNOSIS, OR CAUSE.

Search strategy	Sensitivity[1]	Specificity	Precision
For studies of treatment:			
Clinical trial (pt)	0.93	0.92	0.49
Randomised controlled trial (pt) or Drug therapy (sh) or Therapeutic use (sh) or Random: (tw)	0.99	0.74	0.22
For studies of prognosis:			
Exp cohort studies	0.60	0.80	0.11
Incidence or Exp mortality or Follow up studies or Mortality: (sh) or Prognosis: (tw) or Predict: (tw) or Course (tw)	0.92	0.73	0.11
For studies of aetiology or cause:			
Risk (tw)	0.67	0.79	0.15
Exp cohort studies or Exp risk or Odds and ratio: (tw) or Relative and risk: (tw) or Case and control: (tw)	0.82	0.70	0.14
For studies of diagnosis:			
Diagnosis (pe)	0.80	0.77	0.09
Exp Sensitivity and specificity or Diagnosis: (pe) or Diagnostic use or Sensitivity: (tw) or Specificity: (tw)	0.92	0.73	0.09

[1]**Sensitivity**, as defined in the study on which the table is based, is the proportion of studies in MEDLINE meeting criteria for scientific soundness and clinical relevance that are detected. **Specificity** is the proportion of less sound/relevant studies that are excluded by the search strategy. **Precision** is the proportion of all citations retrieved that are both sound and relevant. (Source: *Evidence-based Medicine*; also see the Web pages.)

Articles

Risk of venous thromboembolism in users of hormone replacement therapy

Edel Daly, Martin P Vessey, Michael M Hawkins, Jeffrey L Carson, Parimala Gough, Sally Marsh

Summary

Background The association between current use of oral contraceptives and increased risk of venous thromboembolism (VTE) has been firmly established. Although data-sheets for hormone replacement therapy (HRT) carry similar warnings as regards VTE, evidence of an association is inconclusive. We carried out a hospital-based case-control study to investigate whether current use of HRT is associated with VTE.

Methods We screened all women aged 45–64 years admitted to hospitals in the area of the Oxford Regional Health Authority with a suspected diagnosis of VTE between February, 1993, and December, 1994. We recruited 81 cases of idiopathic VTE and 146 hospital controls with disorders of eyes, skin, ears, respiratory and alimentary tracts, kidneys, bones, and joints, and trauma; controls were matched to cases for age-group and date and district of admission. To increase the study power, an additional 22 cases of idiopathic VTE and 32 hospital controls admitted before February, 1993, were recruited retrospectively. Participants were questioned about medical and gynaecological history, use of oral contraceptives and HRT, use of other drugs within the previous 3 months, and lifestyle and socioeconomic characteristics. Detailed diagnostic data were extracted from the notes of eligible cases. Matched analyses, adjusted for body-mass index, socioeconomic group, and history of varicose veins, were undertaken by conditional logistic regression.

Findings 44 (42·7%) cases and 44 (24·7%) controls were current users of HRT. The adjusted odds ratio for VTE in current users of HRT compared with non-users (never-users and past users combined) was 3·5 (95% CI 1·8–7·0; p<0·001). No association was found with past use. and risk appeared to be highest among short-term current users (adjusted likelihood ratio test of trend in odds ratios across different durations of current use, p=0·011).

Interpretation Current HRT use is associated with risk of VTE. The increased risk may be concentrated in new users. The number of extra cases appears to be only about one in 5000 users per year. These findings need to be weighed against the probable benefits of long-term treatment, including reductions in risks of osteoporotic fracture and coronary heart disease, and the probable modest increase in risk of breast cancer.

Lancet 1996; **348**: 977–80

See Commentary page 972

University of Oxford, Department of Public Health and Primary Care, Gibson Building, Radcliffe Infirmary, Oxford OX2 6HE, UK
(E Daly BA, Prof M P Vessey MD FRS, J L Carson MD, P Gough BA, S Marsh SRN); **and Childhood Cancer Research Group, Oxford** (M M Hawkins DPhil)

Correspondence to: Ms E Daly

Introduction

Most studies linking the use of oestrogen to increased risk of venous thromboembolism (VTE) have been carried out in young women in relation to use of oral contraceptives.[1] Hormone replacement therapy (HRT) is not generally believed to carry a similar risk in postmenopausal women. Although none of the studies to address this issue has found a significant increase in VTE associated with HRT,[2-5] each lacked power to detect important risks. The *British National Formulary*[6] states that the evidence of an increased thrombotic risk associated with HRT is questionable, but lists active thrombophlebitis or thromboembolic disorders as contraindications to treatment. Similarly, although a working party of the UK Royal College of Obstetricians and Gynaecologists on prophylaxis against thromboembolism concluded that there was insufficient evidence to suggest that HRT is associated with an increased risk of VTE, their report acknowledged the need for further research.[7]

Our study was undertaken to investigate a possible association between current use of HRT and the risk of idiopathic deep-vein thrombosis (DVT) and pulmonary embolism (PE). The protocol was based on that of a case-control study to examine the association between oral-contraceptive use and VTE in young women.[8]

Patients and methods

Cases

Cases were recruited between February, 1993, and December, 1994, from hospitals in the area of the Oxford Regional Health Authority (as defined before April, 1994) by twice-weekly screening of all relevant wards. Eligible cases were women aged 45–64 years with a suspected diagnosis of PE, DVT, or both. Women with a history of PE, DVT, stroke, or myocardial infarction, and those with a history within the previous 6 weeks of surgery, pregnancy, trauma, or illness necessitating bed rest for longer than 1 week were ineligible for inclusion. One case died before she could be interviewed and was excluded.

Detailed diagnostic data were extracted from the notes of eligible cases. On the basis of signs and symptoms and the results of investigations, diagnoses were classified as definite, probable, possible, or other.[5]

PE was classified as definite if established by a ventilation/perfusion scan or angiogram. The classification was probable PE if there was no good evidence of an alternative diagnosis and if any three of the following were reported: haemoptysis; pleuritic chest pain; shortness of breath of sudden onset; syncope with tachypnoea; electrocardiographic (ECG) pattern, chest radiographic changes, or arterial blood gas concentrations compatible with the diagnosis; other compatible clinical signs (pleural rub, raised jugular venous pressure, abnormal heart sounds); compatible perfusion scan or matched defect seen with ventilation/perfusion scan. PE was classified as possible if there was no good evidence of an alternative diagnosis and any two of the nine signs, symptoms, or investigations listed under probable PE were reported.

DVT was classified as definite if venography, duplex scanning, or radioisotope studies confirmed the presence of a DVT. The classification was probable DVT if there was no good evidence of

---

	Cases (n=103)	Controls (n=178)
Age (years)*	53·9 (5·9)	53·9 (5·6)
Number who had undergone hysterectomy	31 (30·1%)	54 (30·3%)
Body-mass index (kg/m²)*	27·6 (5·8)	26·0 (4·6)
Number reporting history of varicose veins	29 (28·2%)	27 (15·2%)
Number reporting history of superficial thrombophlebitis	13 (12·6%)	0
Number who had ever used oral contraceptives	55 (53·4%)	101 (56·7%)
Number who smoked during 3 months before admission	28 (27·2%)	47 (26·6%)
Number in socioeconomic group I or II	23 (22·4%)	57 (32·8%)

*Mean (SD). Smoking status not known for 1 control, body-mass index for 1 case and 2 controls, socioeconomic group for 4 controls.

Table 1: **Characteristics of VTE cases and controls**

an alternative diagnosis, and swelling and induration extended above the knee, and when any two of the following were reported: tenderness on palpation of affected limb; increased superficial temperature of limb; engorgement of superficial veins; doppler ultrasound scan compatible with the diagnosis or equivocal venogram result (the latter was not found in any of our cases). When swelling and induration did not extend above the calf, and in the absence of any other likely cause for the presenting signs and symptoms, a case diagnosis was classified as probable DVT if three of the four signs, symptoms, or investigations listed above were reported. DVT was classified as possible if no good evidence of an alternative diagnosis was reported, and when swelling and induration extended above the knee, and when no more than one of the four signs, symptoms, or investigations listed above was reported. When swelling and induration were confined to the calf, and in the absence of any other likely cause for the presenting signs and symptoms, a case diagnosis was classified as possible if two of the four signs, symptoms, or investigations listed above were reported.

For both PE and DVT, any cases not satisfying any of these criteria were classified as 'other'.

Cases who had diagnoses of both PE and DVT were classified, for the purposes of analysis, to the diagnosis of greater certainty. When both diagnoses were judged equally certain, cases were classified as DVT since this disorder usually precedes PE.

Controls

Controls were recruited from among women admitted to hospital with a diagnosis judged to be unrelated to HRT use in this age-group. Acceptable diagnoses included diseases of the eye, ear, skin, respiratory and alimentary tracts, kidneys, bones, and joints, or trauma. For recruitment, wards were screened in a random order. Up to two controls were recruited per case, matched by 5-year age-group, district of admission, and date of admission (between 2 weeks before and 4 months after the admission date of the corresponding case). The exclusion criteria applied for cases were also applied for controls.

Retrospective recruitment of cases and controls

To increase the study power, additional participants were recruited retrospectively. Details were obtained of all women aged 45–64 years, discharged between April, 1990, and March, 1993, with a first diagnosis of PE or DVT or any of the acceptable control diagnoses, from hospitals in the area of the Oxford Regional Health Authority. Because of financial constraints, only the first 26 such cases (plus 36 matching controls) from Oxford and Kettering were recruited to the study.

Interviews

Participants were interviewed while still in hospital by one of two research nurses. Cases who were discharged before they could be interviewed (23%) were interviewed at home, as were their matched controls. All retrospectively recruited participants were interviewed at home. During the interview the women were questioned about medical and gynaecological history, past and present use of HRT, past and present use of oral contraceptives, use within the past 3 months of other drugs, estimated height and

	n	% of group	
		Current use of HRT	Ever use of HRT
Cases	103	42·7	52·4
Control diagnostic group			
Eye and ear diseases	20	20·0	25·0
Respiratory diseases	16	18·8	37·5
Alimentary diseases	26	23·1	38·5
Renal diseases	18	27·8	44·4
Skin diseases	13	38·5	53·8
Bone and joint disorders	49	22·4	34·7
Hip and wrist fractures	8	37·5	37·5
Other fractures	19	26·3	42·1
Non-fracture trauma	9	22·2	77·8
All controls	178	24·7	39·9

Table 2: **Prevalence of current use and ever use of HRT among cases and control subgroups**

weight, smoking habit, alcohol intake, and occupation. Photographs of currently available HRT and oral-contraceptive preparations were used during the interview to aid recall.

Exclusions

Women were excluded after interview if they reported a history of cancer of the breast, ovary, endometrium, or other recent (diagnosed in the year before the current hospital admission) or active cancer; a history of serious heart disease; or use of anticoagulants or oral contraceptives (four women) in the month before admission. Decisions to exclude were made by an investigator unaware of case or control status and exposure to HRT.

Definitions

Women were classified as current HRT users if they had used the treatment at any time in the month preceding their admission to hospital. One user who did not know the preparation name was included in all analyses except those relating to the type of preparation. Four controls who had stopped using HRT in anticipation of their hospital admission were classified as current users. Tibolone, a synthetic compound with oestrogenic, progestagenic, and androgenic properties, was regarded as HRT, but data for women using this drug are presented separately in the subgroup analyses. Because of evidence of an association between current but not past use of oral contraceptives and risk of VTE,[8] we considered a priori that the most appropriate reference group in all analyses was non-users of HRT (past users and never-users combined), subject to confirmation of no evidence of risk associated with past use in the data from this study. Body-mass index was categorised based on quintiles of control group values. Each woman was assigned to one of six socioeconomic groups based on her partner's occupation, or her own if she was single or if her partner's occupation was not given.[9] Women were classified as current smokers if they had smoked during the 3 months before hospital admission.

Analysis

Conditional logistic regression analyses of matched data[10] were undertaken. Body-mass index, a history of varicose veins, and

Comparison	Cases	Controls	Matched odds ratio (95% CI)	
			Unadjusted	Adjusted*
Relative to never-users				
Never use	49	107	1·0	1·0
Past use	10	27	0·8 (0·4–1·7)	1·1 (0·5–2·6)
Current use	44	44	2·9 (1·5–5·4)	3·6 (1·8–7·3)
Relative to non-users				
Non-use	59	134	1·0	1·0
Current use	44	44	3·0 (1·6–5·6)†	3·5 (1·8–7·0)†

*For body-mass index, history of varicose veins, and socioeconomic group.
†Likelihood ratio test of a difference in risk of VTE between non-users and current users of HRT, p<0·001.

Table 3: **Odds ratios of VTE in relation to current HRT use**

socioeconomic group were judged a priori to be potential confounding variables and were included in adjusted models if they produced a change of at least 5% in the estimated odds ratio of VTE associated with HRT.[11]

Results

108 cases (69 with DVT and 39 with PE) and 232 controls satisfied all inclusion criteria. The proportions of cases with definite, probable, possible, and other diagnostic certainty ratings were 73%, 20%, 4%, and 3% for DVT, and 33%, 51%, 10%, and 5% for PE. Cases in the 'other' category were excluded from all further analyses. Participants without matching cases or controls were also excluded. 103 cases and 178 controls remained; of these, 22 cases and 32 controls had been recruited retrospectively. The characteristics of the study population are given in table 1. As expected, mean body-mass index was higher among cases than controls, reflecting the increased risk of VTE in overweight people. Higher proportions of cases than controls reported histories of varicose veins and superficial thrombophlebitis, whereas a lower proportion were classified in the higher socioeconomic groups.

Overall 44 (42·7%) cases and 44 (24·7%) controls were current users of HRT (table 2). A matched analysis yielded an odds ratio for VTE associated with current HRT use of 3·0 (95% CI 1·6–5·6) compared with non-users (never-users and past users combined; table 3). Each of the potential confounding variables (body-mass index, a history of varicose veins, and socioeconomic group) produced a change of at least 5% in the estimated risk of VTE associated with HRT.[11] After adjustment for these factors, the odds ratio was 3·5 (1·8–7·0).

Estimated odds ratios in relation to duration of current episode of use are shown in table 4. The odds ratios

associated with short-term use of HRT are higher than those for longer durations, and this effect was strengthened somewhat by adjustment for confounding. There was evidence that the logarithms of the odds ratios decreased linearly with increasing duration of current use; the adjusted likelihood ratio test for such an effect yielded a p value of 0·011. Risk estimates according to oestrogen dose, type of preparation, and route of delivery are also shown in table 4. Among current users, there was no significant difference in the risk of VTE between high-dose and low-dose preparations, between oral and transdermal therapy, or between unopposed oestrogen and combined oestrogen-progestagen therapy.

In analyses by certainty of case diagnosis the unadjusted estimated odds ratios for VTE associated with current HRT use were higher for the definite (2·9 [95% CI 1·3–6·5]) and probable (4·7 [1·3–17·4]) categories, than for the possible (1·4 [0·3–7·5]) category. Various multivariate analyses were undertaken to investigate the effects of exclusion of women with certain characteristics that might lead to biased results. There were no important differences in the odds ratios associated with current HRT use, or in the pattern in relation to duration of current use, when we excluded all women with a history of superficial thrombophlebitis; controls with an index diagnosis of fracture; cases with a diagnostic rating of probable or possible; and retrospectively recruited participants. However, in the last two subgroup analyses, we were unable to obtain risk estimates relating to duration of use, since there were too few data for a regression equation to be fitted.

Discussion

The results of our study and those of Jick and colleagues[12] suggest a possible causal relation between current HRT use and idiopathic VTE. This interpretation is supported by results from a study of exogenous hormones in relation to risk of PE by Grodstein and colleagues.[13] In our study, risk of VTE seemed to be highest among short-term users, whereas no association was seen with past use. Although the magnitude of estimated risk was greater among users of higher-dose preparations than among users of lower-dose preparations, this difference was not significant. Similarly, we found no significant difference in risk between users of oral and transdermal therapy, or between users of unopposed oestrogen and combined oestrogen-progestagen therapy.

At least three case-control studies and one small clinical trial have investigated the possible association between HRT and VTE.[2–5] The sample sizes ranged between 17 and 121 cases, and the studies found non-significant relative risks between 0·7 and 1·8. In each, no more than six cases had been exposed to HRT, whereas our results are based on 44 HRT-exposed cases. In the clinical trial,[4] no cases of serious embolic disease occurred among 84 long-term hospital inpatients treated with HRT for 10 years, whereas one case of VTE occurred among the untreated group. The largest study to date found a relative risk of 0·79 (95% CI 0·30–2·08).[5] However, VTE had occurred while the women were in hospital for another reason in more than a third of cases, 21% of cases had a history of previous VTE, and the average age of the participants was high (65 years).

Preferential referral and diagnosis of exposed cases is a potential source of bias in observational studies.[14] Analysis

Comparison	Cases	Controls	Matched odds ratio (95% CI)	
			Unadjusted	Adjusted*
Non-users†	59	134	1·0	1·0
Duration of current episode of use (months)				
1–12	14	10	4·1 (1·5–10·8)	6·7 (2·1–21·3)
13–36	16	12	3·2 (1·4–7·5)	4·4 (1·6–11·9)
37–60	4	11	1·2 (0·3–4·5)	1·9 (0·5–7·8)
⩾61	10	11	2·7 (1·0–7·2)	2·1 (0·8–6·1)
Composition of HRT‡				
Oestrogen only	22	21	3·1 (1·4–6·5)	3·2 (1·4–7·4)
Oestrogen and progestagen	20	20	4·0 (1·6–9·6)	5·3 (1·9–14·6)
Tibolone	1	3	0·6 (0·1–6·4)	1·1 (0·1–13·0·
Oestrogen dose§				
Lower-dose oestrogen	17	14	4·1 (1·7–10·0)	3·7 (1·3–10·2)
Higher-dose oestrogen	16	16	3·4 (1·4–8·4)	6·6 (2·2–19·6)
Unknown dose	9	10	2·6 (0·9–7·4)	2·4 (0·8–7·1)
Implant	1	1	5·1 (0·3–88·9)	2·3 (0·1–65·6)
Tibolone	1	3	0·6 (0·1–6·2)	1·2 (0·1–14·3)
Route of administration				
Oral therapy	37	32	3·6 (1·8–7·2)	4·6 (2·1–10·1)
Transdermal therapy	5	8	2·2 (0·7–7·5)	2·0 (0·5–7·6)
Implant	1	1	3·9 (0·2–66·4)	2·1 (0·1–50·2)
Tibolone	1	3	0·6 (0·1–6·6)	1·1 (0·1–13·2)

*For body-mass index, history of varicose veins, and socioeconomic group.
†Never-users and past users, baseline category throughout. ‡Unknown for 1 case.
§Lower dose includes oral preparations containing 0·625 mg conjugated equine oestrogens, 1 mg oestradiol/oestradiol valerate, or 1·5 mg piperazine oestrone sulphate; and includes transdermal preparations delivering 50 μg oestradiol per 24 h. Higher dose includes oral preparations containing 1·25 mg conjugated equine oestrogens or 2 mg oestradiol/oestradiol valerate; and includes transdermal preparations delivering 100 μg oestradiol per 24 h.

Table 4: **Odds ratios of VTE in relation to current HRT use by duration of current episode of use, type of preparation, oestrogen dose, and route of administration**

by certainty of case diagnosis in our study yielded risk estimates that were lowest in the possible category for both DVT and PE; the confidence intervals were wide, however, because of small numbers in these subgroups. Exclusion of cases without a definite diagnosis did not reveal any appreciable differences in the risk estimates associated with HRT use.

The problem of recall bias is a common criticism of case-control studies. Since the exposure of interest in this study was use of HRT in the month before admission, we would expect very little recall bias among prospectively recruited subjects, most of whom were interviewed while still in hospital. Although recall bias might be of some concern in relation to the participants who were recruited retrospectively (20%), use of photographs of packets of all available HRT preparations during the interview should have aided recall. In addition, the relative risk of VTE in association with current HRT use was essentially unchanged when the retrospectively recruited subjects were excluded.

The use of hospital patients as controls in epidemiological studies of postmenopausal oestrogen has been criticised, since such women may be less likely to be using HRT; however, prevalence of use among controls in this study was similar to that among women attending for breast screening in Oxfordshire.[15]

15% of controls recruited to this study were patients who had sustained fractures. Although women with osteoporotic fracture may be less likely to have used HRT,[16] a previous diagnosis of osteoporosis might increase their chances of treatment. Of the controls with fractures, less than a third had fractures of the hip, wrist, or vertebrae, types that may indicate underlying osteoporosis. None had a previous diagnosis of osteoporosis and the proportion using HRT did not differ significantly from that in other controls (table 2). Exclusion of all controls with an index diagnosis of fracture from our analyses did not materially change the results.

A history of previous DVT or PE was an exclusion criterion. However, a significantly higher proportion of cases than of controls reported a history of thrombophlebitis (table 1). Treatment prescribed for past episodes of thrombophlebitis included antibiotics and non-steroidal anti-inflammatory drugs rather than anticoagulants, which suggests that the thrombophlebitis was superficial rather than deep. 54% of these women had ever used HRT, compared with 44% of all other women; the proportions for current use were 46% and 31%, respectively. These findings suggest that doctors do not generally regard a history of superficial thrombophlebitis as a contraindication to HRT. Our results did not change substantially when women with a history of thrombophlebitis were omitted from the analysis.

On the basis of these results and on regional population statistics,[17] the annual rate of idiopathic VTE per 100 000 women aged 45–64 years is estimated to be 27·4 among HRT users and 10·9 among non-users, which gives an annual total of 16·5 cases per 100 000 that may be attributed to HRT. This risk may be entirely acceptable to women using HRT in the short-term for the relief of menopausal symptoms, especially to those without other risk factors for VTE. For long-term HRT users, these findings need to be weighed against the probable benefits of long-term treatment, including reductions in risks of osteoporotic fracture[16] and coronary heart disease,[18,19] and the probable slight increase in risk of breast cancer.[20] Since mortality from venous thromboembolism is low, our findings are unlikely to change the overall balance of benefits and risks of long-term treatment substantially.[21] Further research is needed to establish whether HRT is contraindicated in the presence of other risk factors for venous thromboembolism, including obesity, recent surgery, immobilisation, and thrombophilic disorders.

We thank Schering Health Care Ltd, Novo Nordisk Pharmaceuticals, and the Knott Family Trust for their financial support of this work. MPV holds a research consultancy with Novo Nordisk Pharmaceuticals. JLC was a Fogarty Senior International Fellow at the University of Oxford.

References

1 Vessey M, Mant D, Smith A, Yeates D. Oral contraceptives and venous thromboembolism: findings in a large prospective study. *BMJ* 1986; **292:** 526.

2 The Boston Collaborative Drug Surveillance Program. Surgically confirmed gallbladder disease, venous thromboembolism and breast tumors in relation to postmenopausal estrogen therapy. *N Engl J Med* 1974; **290:** 15–19.

3 Petitti DB, Wingerd J, Pellegrin F, Ramcharan S. Risk of vascular disease in women. *JAMA* 1979; **242:** 1150–54.

4 Nachtigall LE, Nachtigall RH, Nachtigall RD, Beckman EM. Estrogen replacement therapy II: a prospective study in the relationship to carcinoma and cardiovascular and metabolic problems. *Obstet Gynecol* 1979; **54:** 74–79.

5 Devor M, Barrett-Connor E, Renvall M, Feigal D, Ramsdell J. Estrogen replacement therapy and the risk of venous thrombosis. *Am J Med* 1992; **92:** 275–82.

6 British National Formulary Number 28. London: British Medical Association and the Royal Pharmaceutical Society of Great Britain, 1995.

7 Report of the RCOG Working Party on Prophylaxis against Thromboembolism in Gynaecology and Obstetrics. London: Chameleon Press, 1995.

8 World Health Organization Collaborative Study of Cardiovascular Disease and Steroid Hormone Contraception. Venous thromboembolic disease and combined oral contraceptives: results of international multicentre case-control study. *Lancet* 1995; **346:** 1575–82.

9 OPCS. Standard occupational classification, volumes 1–3. London: HM Stationery Office, 1990.

10 Breslow NE, Day NE. Statistical methods in cancer research I: analysis of case-control studies. Lyon: International Agency for Research on Cancer, 1980: 192–246.

11 Maldonado G, Greenland S. Simulation study of confounder-selection strategies. *Am J Epidemiol* 1993; **138:** 923–36.

12 Jick H, Derby LE, Wald Myers M, Vasilakis C, Newton KM. Risk of hospital admission for idiopathic venous thromboembolism among users of postmenopausal oestrogens. *Lancet* 1996; **348:** 981–83.

13 Grodstein F, Stampfer MJ, Goldhaber SZ, et al. Prospective study of exogenous hormones and risk of pulmonary embolism in women. *Lancet* 1996; **348:** 983–87.

14 Realini JP, Goldzieher JW. Oral contraceptives and cardiovascular disease: a critique of the epidemiological studies. *Am J Obstet Gynecol* 1985; **152:** 729–98.

15 Banks E, Crossley B, English R, Richardson A. Women doctors' use of hormone replacement therapy: high prevalence of use is not confined to doctors. *BMJ* 1996; **312:** 638.

16 Compston JE. HRT and osteoporosis. *Br Med Bull* 1992; **48:** 309–44.

17 OPCS. 1993-based subpopulation projections. Series PP3, no 9, table 5. London: HM Stationery Office, 1995.

18 Grodstein F, Stampfer M. The epidemiology of coronary heart disease and estrogen replacement in postmenopausal women. *Prog Cardiovasc Dis* 1995; **38:** 199–210.

19 The Writing Group for the PEPI Trial. Effects of estrogen or estrogen/progestin regimens on heart disease risk factors in postmenopausal women: the Postmenopausal Estrogen/Progestin Interventions Trial. *JAMA* 1995; **273:** 199–208.

20 Grady D, Rubin SM, Petitti DB, et al. Hormone therapy to prevent disease and prolong life in postmenopausal women. *Ann Intern Med* 1992; **117:** 1016–37.

21 Daly E, Vessey MP, Barlow D, Gray A, McPherson K, Roche M. Hormone replacement therapy in a risk-benefit perspective. *Maturitas* 1996; **23:** 247–59.

Citation:

Are the results of this harm study valid?

Were there clearly defined groups of patients, similar in all important ways other than exposure to the treatment or other cause?

Were treatment exposures and clinical outcomes measured the same ways in both groups, e.g. was the assessment of outcomes either objective (death) or blinded to exposure?

Was the follow-up of study patients complete and long enough?

Do the results satisfy some 'diagnostic tests for causation'?

- Is it clear that the exposure preceded the onset of the outcome?

- Is there a dose-response gradient?

- Is there positive evidence from a 'dechallenge–rechallenge' study?

- Is the association consistent from study to study?

- Does the association make biological sense?

Are the valid results from this harm study important?

		Adverse Outcome		Totals
		Present (case)	**Absent (control)**	
Exposed to the Treatment	Yes (cohort)	a	b	a+b
	No (cohort)	c	d	c+d
	Totals	a+c	b+d	a+b+c+d

In a randomised trial or cohort study: relative risk = RR = [a/(a+b)]/[c/(c+d)]
In a case-control study: odds ratio (or relative odds) = OR = ad/bc
In this study:

Should these valid, potentially important results of a critical appraisal about a harmful treatment change the treatment of your patient?

Can the study results be extrapolated to your patient?

What are your patient's risks of the adverse outcome?
To calculate the NNH[1] for any odds ratio (OR) and
your patient's expected event rate for this adverse
event if they were **not** exposed to this treatment (PEER):

$$NNH = \frac{PEER\ (OR - 1) + 1}{PEER\ (OR - 1) \times (1 - PEER)}$$

What are your patient's preferences, concerns and
expectations from this treatment?

What alternative treatments are available?

Additional notes

[1] The number of patients you need to treat to harm one of them.

Citation: Daly E *et al.* (1996) Risk of venous thromboembolism in users of hormone replacement therapy. *Lancet.* **348**(9033): 977–80.

Are the results of this harm study valid?

Were there clearly defined groups of patients, similar in all important ways other than exposure to the treatment or other cause?	**Yes. Cases were women admitted to hospital with a diagnosis of deep vein thrombosis or pulmonary embolism. Controls were women matched by age, district and date of admission, who were admitted to hospital with diagnoses unlikely to be affected by use of hormone replacement therapy (HRT).**
Were treatment exposures and clinical outcomes measured the same ways in both groups, e.g. was the assessment of outcomes either objective (death) or blinded to exposure?	**Yes. HRT use was ascertained by interviews with a research nurse who had photographs of the medications to assist recall. The assessment of outcomes was based on pre-specified clinical criteria, although it was unclear whether the assessment was blinded. Because this was a case-control study, the problem of recall bias must be considered, but is likely to have been minimal.**
Was the follow-up of study patients complete and long enough?	**This was a case-control study. The subjects were therefore not followed through time.**

Do the results satisfy some 'diagnostic tests for causation'?

• Is it clear that the exposure preceded the onset of the outcome?	**Yes.**
• Is there a dose-response gradient?	**Yes, the risk was higher with higher doses and longer duration of HRT.**
• Is there positive evidence from a 'dechallenge–rechallenge' study?	**No.**
• Is the association consistent from study to study?	**When we reviewed the abstract of the accompanying paper by Jick *et al.* the results were very similar.**
• Does the association make biological sense?	**Yes, there has been long-standing concern that oestrogens may affect the clotting system.**

Are the valid results from this harm study important?

		Venous thromboembolism		Totals
		Present (case)	Absent (control)	
Exposed to HRT	Yes (cohort)	44 a	44 b	a+b
	No (cohort)	59 c	134 d	c+d
	Totals	103 a+c	178 b+d	a+b+c+d

In this study: odds ratio = 44 x 134/44 x 59 = 2.3. Because the cases and controls were matched on certain variables, the authors used a matched analysis which yielded a slightly different odds ratio of 3.0 (95% CI 1.6–5.6). After controlling for other factors that might influence the risk of DVT, the odds ratio rose to 3.5 (1.8–7.0).

Should these valid, potentially important results of a critical appraisal about a harmful treatment change the treatment of your patient?

Can the study results be extrapolated to your patient?

Bias is a potential problem with case-control studies. However, the study has been well conducted, and is consistent with the other reported study of this association which you have identified. Until other evidence comes along, we should assume that HRT does increase the risk of DVT. Interestingly, as we went to press, a randomised trial of HRT use (see below for reference) reported a similar risk of DVT, adding strong confirmation of the finding.

What are your patient's risks of the adverse outcome?
To calculate the NNH[1] for any odds ratio (OR) and your patient's expected event rate for this adverse event if they were **not** exposed to this treatment (PEER):

$$NNH = \frac{PEER \, (OR - 1) + 1}{PEER \, (OR - 1) \times (1 - PEER)}$$

The odds ratio tells you how much greater the risk is in those who take HRT compared to those who don't. To make clinical sense of this, you need to know the absolute risk faced by someone who does not take HRT.

On the basis of population statistics, the paper suggests that the annual rate of DVT in women age 45–64 who do not use HRT is about 11/100,000 (0.00011). If the odds ratio is 3.5, then the NNH, using the formula, is 3638. Given this patient's past history she is probably at greater risk. If you consider her risk to be double then the NNH would become 3638/2 = 1819.

[1] The number of patients you need to treat to harm one of them.

What are your patient's preferences, concerns and expectations from this treatment?	**This is the critical factor in the decision whether to prescribe. She may wish to accept the small risk of another DVT depending how she views her symptoms.**
What alternative treatments are available?	**No treatment is obviously an option as some of her symptoms may improve with time.**

Additional notes

1 The fact that the odds ratio actually increased when potentially confounding factors were taken into account, strengthens the case that it is a true association.

2 Similar results have recently been found in a randomised trial:

Hulley S, Grady D, Bush T *et al.* for the HERS Research Group (1998) Randomized trial of estrogen plus progestin for secondary prevention of coronary heart disease in postmenopausal women. *JAMA.* **280:** 605–13.

CAT – HORMONE REPLACEMENT THERAPY (HRT) INCREASES THE RISK OF VENOUS THROMBOEMBOLISM IN POST-MENOPAUSAL WOMEN

Appraised by Tim Lancaster.
Expiry date: 2000.

Clinical Bottom Line

HRT increases the risk of DVT about three-fold. However, for women at average risk, the increase in absolute risk is small.

Citation

Daly E, Vessey MP, Hawkins MM *et al*. (1996) Risk of venous thromboembolism in users of hormone replacement therapy. *Lancet*. **348**(9033): 977–80.

Clinical Question

In post-menopausal women does HRT lead to an increased risk of deep vein thrombosis, and if so, what is the size of the risk?

Search Terms

In MEDLINE 'Thromboembolism' (MeSH), 'HRT' and 'risk' (text words).

The Study

A case-control study among women aged 45–64 admitted to hospitals in the area of Oxford Regional Health Authority. All women with a suspected diagnosis of venous thromboembolism over a specified time period were identified. If they met pre-specified criteria for diagnosis, they were classified as cases. Controls were women admitted to hospital with disorders not related to HRT use, matched to cases by age-group, date and district of admission. Cases and controls were questioned about medical and gynaecological history, use of oral contraceptives and HRT, uses of other drugs within the previous three months, and lifestyle and socioeconomic characteristics.

The Evidence

		Venous thromboembolism		Totals
		Present (case)	**Absent (control)**	
Exposed to HRT	Yes (cohort)	44 a	44 b	a+b
	No (cohort)	59 c	134 d	c+d
	Totals	103 a+c	178 b+d	a+b+c+d

In this study: odds ratio = 44 x 134/44 x 59 = 2.3. Because the cases and controls were matched on certain variables, the authors used a matched analysis which yielded a slightly different odds ratio of 3.0 (95% CI 1.6–5.6). After controlling for other factors that might influence the risk of DVT, the odds ratio rose to 3.5 (1.8–7.0).

The absolute risk of DVT in post-menopausal women is quite small, about 10/100,000 women per year. We calculated the number needed to harm at about 3,600.

Comments

1 Because of possible bias in case-control studies, a relative risk of 3.0, even if statistically significant, might be considered inconclusive. However, in this case the finding was consistent with another study conducted in a similar population, and was subsequently confirmed in a randomised trial.

2 The absolute increase in risk of DVT with HRT is small and the NNH is therefore large. Our patient had a past history of DVT, so her absolute risk may be higher.

Other useful references

Jick H, Derby LE, Myers MW *et al.* (1996) Risk of hospital admission for idiopathic venous thromboembolism among users of postmenopausal oestrogens. *Lancet.* **348**(9033): 981–3

Hulley S, Grady D, Bush T *et al.* for the HERS Research Group (1998) Randomized trial of estrogen plus progestin for secondary prevention of coronary heart disease in postmenopausal women. *JAMA.* **280:** 605–13.

PART

A | Critical appraisal of a systematic review

You have performed an audit of antibiotic prescription for acute respiratory infection in your six-partner practice. This has shown that rates of prescribing of antibiotics for cough vary significantly between the partners. Your partners agree to review practice prescribing policy. You volunteer to report a summary of the evidence on prescribing for acute cough, as the first step to agreeing standards that will form the basis of the practice policy. You form the clinical question: 'In patients presenting with acute cough in general practice, do antibiotics lead to reduction in symptoms (and/or increase in side-effects) compared to symptomatic treatments alone.'

You do a MEDLINE search using the words 'antibiotic' and 'cough', and retrieve 71 articles. Adding in the term 'systematic review' reduces the yield to one article, which you select for appraisal: *BMJ* (1998) **316**: 906–10.

Read the systematic review and decide:
1   Is the evidence from this systematic review valid?
2   Is this valid evidence from this systematic review important?
3   Can you apply this valid and important evidence from this systematic review to guide your practice policy in this area?

If you want to read some strategies for answering these sorts of questions, you could have a look at pp 97–9, 140–1 and 166–72 in *Evidence-based Medicine*.

PART

B | Searching for evidence in the Cochrane Library

We show you how to search the Cochrane Library, an electronic database of systematic reviews done by the Cochrane Collaboration, abstracts of other systematic reviews from the world literature, citations from several hundred thousand randomised trials and information about the Cochrane Collaboration.

To help us organise your presentations for Sessions 6 and 7, please complete and hand in the form on the next page.

CASE
PRESENTATION

My tentative clinical question:

My name: _____

Contact address: _____

Contact phone number: _____

Bleep: _____

E-mail: _____

General practice

Quantitative systematic review of randomised controlled trials comparing antibiotic with placebo for acute cough in adults

Tom Fahey, Nigel Stocks, Toby Thomas

Toby Thomas died
in a road traffic
accident on
25 November 1996

Division of Primary
Care, University of
Bristol, Canynge
Hall, Bristol
BS8 2PR
Tom Fahey,
senior lecturer

Nigel Stocks,
clinical lecturer

United Medical and
Dental Schools of
Guy's and St
Thomas's Hospitals,
London SE11 6SP
Toby Thomas,
medical student

Correspondence to:
Dr Fahey
tom.fahey@bris.ac.uk

BMJ 1998;316:906–10

Abstract

Objectives: To assess whether antibiotic treatment for acute cough is effective and to measure the side effects of such treatment.

Design: Quantitative systematic review of randomised placebo controlled trials.

Data sources: Nine trials (8 published, 1 unpublished) retrieved from a systematic search (electronic databases, contact with authors, contact with drug manufacturers, reference lists); no restriction on language.

Main outcome measures: Proportion of subjects with productive cough at follow up (7-11 days after consultation with general practitioner); proportion of subjects who had not improved clinically at follow up; proportion of subjects who reported side effects from taking antibiotic or placebo.

Results: Eight trials contributed to the meta-analysis. Resolution of cough was not affected by antibiotic treatment (relative risk 0.85 (95% confidence interval 0.73 to 1.00)), neither was clinical improvement at re-examination (relative risk 0.62 (0.36 to 1.09)). The side effects of antibiotic were more common in the antibiotic group when compared to placebo (relative risk 1.51 (0.86 to 2.64)).

Conclusions: Treatment with antibiotic does not affect the resolution of cough or alter the course of illness. The benefits of antibiotic treatment are marginal for most patients with acute cough and may be outweighed by the side effects of treatment.

Introduction

Acute cough and respiratory tract infection are terms used to describe a wide variety of clinical syndromes. Symptoms range from cough without sputum to an illness characterised by expectoration of mucopurulent sputum, fever, general malaise, and dyspnoea,[1] but coughing is nearly always present.[1-4] Therefore, although the terms acute bronchitis, upper respiratory tract infection, common cold, and chest infection are used in a clinical context to define separate disease entities, they represent a range of respiratory tract infection whose symptoms, causative agents, and resolution vary.[1 2]

Acute cough is a common reason for consulting a general practitioner. The fourth national morbidity survey in the United Kingdom found that the overall consultation rate for acute upper respiratory infections (code 465 of the international classification of diseases, ninth revision (ICD-9)) and acute bronchitis and bronchiolitis (ICD-9 code 466) was 772 and 719 per 10 000 person years at risk.[5]

The clinical syndrome of cough is nearly always preceded and associated with a viral nasopharyngitis.[1 2] The causes of such infection are usually influenza virus, para-influenza virus, respiratory syncytial virus, rhinovirus, coronavirus, and adenovirus.[2 6 7] Infection with non-viral organisms such as *Bordetella pertussis*, *Mycoplasma pneumoniae*, and *Chlamydia pneumonia* may also occur, some studies reporting a high prevalence of infection with *Mycoplasma* spp, particularly in young adults.[7 8] Secondary bacterial infection occurs in a certain proportion of cases, usually with *Haemophilus influenzae* and *Streptococcus pneumoniae*.[1 2 7] Because bacteria are carried as normal resident flora in the upper respiratory tract, the aetiological role of bacteria cultured from sputum samples is unclear.[2] In a study based in the United Kingdom 25% of sputum culture samples from people being treated for acute bronchitis grew recognised or potential respiratory bacterial pathogens.[9] A community based longitudinal study in the United Kingdom showed that a potential pathogen was cultured in only 29% of cases, with viruses being identified more frequently than *Mycoplasma* spp and bacteria being identified least of all.[4] In a community based study in the United Kingdom of 206 patients with more severe respiratory tract infection (inclusion criteria were productive cough, focal signs on chest examination, and prescription of antibiotic) an aetiological diagnosis was established in 91 (44%) patients.[10] The most commonly identified pathogens were *S pneumoniae* (36%), *H influenzae* (10%), and influenza viruses (13%).[10] An accompanying editorial highlighted the difficulty in clinically differentiating between the more severe forms of bronchitis and pneumonia in the community.[11]

Microbiological investigation of acute bronchitis is rare in general practice.[1 9 12] Differentiation between viral and bacterial infection is difficult on the basis of symptoms alone,[1] and therefore general practitioners

906

have substantially different diagnostic and treatment thresholds for respiratory tract infection in the community.[1][12][13]

Concern about the treatment of acute cough with antibiotics is not new.[14][15] Review articles have questioned the value of antibiotic treatment for acute bronchitis and related conditions.[1][16-19] To our knowledge, the absolute risk of illness without antibiotic treatment, the likely benefits and risks of treatment, and the balance of risk and benefit for individual patients have not been measured. We therefore carried out a systematic review of randomised controlled trials to establish whether antibiotics are effective in the treatment of acute cough in the community.

Methods

Inclusion and exclusion criteria
We included studies of patients aged greater than 12 years who were attending a family practice clinic, community based outpatient department, or an outpatient department attached to a hospital. We included patients who complained of acute cough with or without purulent sputum that had not been treated in the preceding week with antibiotic. Patients with chronic obstructive airways disease were excluded. The included studies were prospective trials in which antibiotic was allocated by formal randomisation or by quasi-randomisation, such as alternate allocation to treatment and placebo groups. Only placebo controlled trials were included; comparative studies between different classes of antibiotics were excluded. Categorical and continuous outcomes were reported in the randomised controlled trials identified at the start of the review.[20-28] Many different outcomes were reported in individual randomised controlled trials; we concentrated on the three most commonly reported outcomes: the proportion of subjects reporting productive cough, the proportion of subjects who had not improved clinically at re-examination, and the proportion of subjects who reported side effects from taking antibiotic or placebo.

Systematic search
We searched Medline and EMBASE databases from 1966 and 1982 respectively using the recommended Cochrane Collaboration search strategy[20] and the medical subject heading (MeSH) terms "cough," "bronchitis," "sputum," and "respiratory tract infections." The search was not restricted to the English language. We also searched for references from published research by using the Science Citation Index and searching references in published studies and abstracts, particularly for those published before 1966. We conducted a search on the Controlled Trials Register from the Cochrane Library[30] with the search terms "bronchitis," "chest infection," and "common cold." We contacted authors of published trials requesting knowledge of any unpublished studies. We also wrote to drug companies in the United Kingdom that manufacture antibiotics (as given in the *British National Formulary*) requesting unpublished trials.

Assessment of quality and extraction of data
Each trial was read independently by TF and NS, who then assessed the quality of each study according to the

four criteria outlined in the *Cochrane Collaboration Handbook*.[31] Each criterion—selection bias, performance bias, attrition bias, and detection bias—was scored from 1 to 3, so the highest score for an individual trial was 12. Measurement of agreement between reviewers was calculated by means of the kappa statistic and disagreement resolved by consensus. Data were extracted independently; when data were missing or incomplete we contacted the authors of the trial for clarification.

Analysis
Because the events in the treatment and control arms occurred frequently, significance and clinical importance were evaluated by estimating relative risk.[32] We explored differences in baseline risk and heterogeneity between studies by using L'Abbe plots (see fig 1).[33] As the inclusion criteria and event rates reported in the control arms varied, the pooled relative risks were estimated with 95% confidence intervals by means of both random effects and fixed effects models.[34] Antibiotic is significantly better than placebo in improving a condition when the upper limit of the 95% confidence interval is < 1. Conversely, side effects of antibiotic treatment are significant when the lower 95% confidence limit of the relative risk is > 1.

Relative risks were calculated with REVMAN 3.0 (Update Software 1996). We calculated the numbers needed to treat with a spreadsheet (Microsoft EXCEL 5.0).[35]

Results

Trials found
Our search uncovered nine trials that met the inclusion criteria for this review (M Stephenson, unpublished

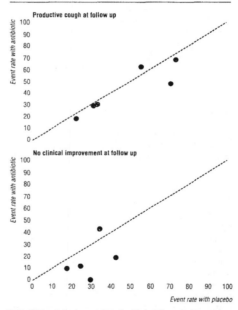

Fig 1 L'Abbe plots of proportion of subjects with productive cough at follow up at 7-11 days (six trials) and of proportion of subjects who had not improved clinically at 7-11 days (five trials)

BMJ VOLUME 316   21 MARCH 1998

907

data).[21-28] The losses to follow up, antibiotic regimen, outcome measured, recommendation for antibiotic treatment, and characteristics of patients for these nine trials are available as two tables on the *BMJ*'s website (www.bmj.com).

We excluded Howie and Clark's trial from the 1970s in 829 patients.[29] Although the unit of randomisation was patients who were instructed to take either antibiotic or placebo at the start of a respiratory illness, the unit of analysis was episodes of illness. Some patients did not contribute any episodes of illness to the analysis (198/829 participants, or 24% of those randomised) while others reported more than one episode of illness (1.52 and 1.55 courses in the antibiotic and placebo arms respectively).[29] This trial reported no difference between antibiotic and placebo in all outcomes reported at the end of the trial. One other unpublished trial that had reported no difference in outcome between antibiotic and placebo in 33 patients,[36] had no original data remaining (S Thomas, personal communication). Franks and Gleiner reported the average percentage of days with cough over a period of seven days (all subjects in placebo arm, 92% of subjects in antibiotic arm) but not the number of patients with cough at a specified end point.[32] No further data were available (P Franks, personal communication), so this trial contributed data to the part of the meta-analysis which examined the side effects of treatment only. King et al included patients aged 8 years and over, but the average age of participants was 37 years and so we included this trial.[27] Finally, one trial by Scherl et al did not contribute data

to the meta-analysis because it reported on a continuous variable, the mean number of days with cough.[28] No additional information could be obtained because the author of the report had died.

This left us with a total of eight trials reporting on the three specified outcome measures. We excluded several trials we judged to be inadequately randomised, case series of early antibiotic use, three trials of the common cold, and eleven trials in children (references available on website (www.bmj.com)). A subgroup of 75 patients with tracheobronchitis from a trial with the diagnostic label of the common cold (L Kaiser, personal communication) was included in a sensitivity analysis on the outcome of resolution of illness.[37]

Assessment of quality

The kappa scores for agreement between reviewers for each of the four variables measuring the quality of trials were 0.5 (moderate agreement) for selection, 0.57 (moderate agreement) for performance, 0.85 (substantial agreement) for attrition, and 1 (almost perfect agreement) for blinding. The overall kappa for trial quality was 0.54 (moderate agreement).

Baseline risk and diagnosis

The six trials that reported resolution of productive cough as an outcome measure had varied considerably in this measure (fig 1) (M Stephenson, unpublished data).[21 23 25-27] Such differences highlight the range of illness and the differences between trials in diagnosis of acute cough. However, the five trials that had outcome data on the course of clinical improvement were similar in the reported resolution of illness (fig 1).[21 23-26]

Proportion of subjects with productive cough at follow up

Study	Antibiotic	Placebo	Relative risk (95% CI) random effects model	Weight (%)	Relative risk (95% CI) random effects model
Dunlay et al[25]	10/21	17/24		9.6	0.67 (0.40 to 1.13)
King et al[27]	28/41	27/31		41.3	0.78 (0.61 to 1.01)
Stephenson (unpublished)	24/81	27/82		12.3	0.90 (0.57 to 1.42)
Stott and West[21]	30/104	32/103		14.7	0.93 (0.61 to 1.41)
Verheij et al[26]	13/72	16/72		6.0	0.81 (0.42 to 1.56)
Williamson[23]	23/37	18/32		16.3	1.11 (0.74 to 1.64)
Total (95% CI)	128/356	137/344		100.0	0.85 (0.73 to 1.00)
$\chi^2 = 3.21$, df=5, Z=1.94					

0.1 0.2   1   5 10
Favours antibiotic   Favours placebo

Fig 2 Comparison of antibiotic and placebo treatment on resolution of productive cough at days 7-11

Proportion of subjects who had not improved clinically at follow up

Study	Antibiotic	Placebo	Relative risk (95% CI) random effects model	Weight (%)	Relative risk (95% CI) random effects model
Brickfield et al[24]	5/26	10/24		19.6	0.46 (0.18 to 1.16)
Dunlay et al[25]	0/23	6/21		3.6	0.07 (0.00 to 1.18)
Stott and West[21]	10/104	17/103		24.4	0.58 (0.28 to 1.21)
Verheij et al[26]	9/73	17/72		24.2	0.52 (0.25 to 1.09)
Williamson[23]	16/37	11/32		28.2	1.26 (0.69 to 2.30)
Total (95% CI)	40/263	61/252		100.0	0.62 (0.36 to 1.09)
$\chi^2 = 8.21$, df=4, Z=1.66					

0.1 0.2   1   5 10
Favours antibiotic   Favours placebo

Fig 3 Comparison of antibiotic and placebo treatment on clinical improvement at days 7-11

Efficacy of antibiotic

Antibiotic treatment was no better than placebo when the resolution of cough at days 7-11 was assessed (relative risk 0.85 (95% confidence interval 0.73 to 1.00)) (fig 2). Similarly, when the proportion of subjects who had not improved clinically was assessed at days 7-11 in five trials antibiotic treatment did not significantly improve the resolution of illness (relative risk 0.62 (0.36 to 1.09)) (fig 3).[21 23-26] Inclusion of a subgroup of 75 patients with tracheobronchitis in a trial of the common cold who were randomly allocated to co-amoxiclav or placebo[37] did not alter the pooled results for resolution of illness (relative risk 0.71 (0.43 to 1.18), χ^2 test for heterogeneity = 16.87, df = 5, P < 0.5).

Side effects of treatment

The mean percentage of subjects reporting side effects from antibiotic treatment in seven trials was 19% (range 12% to 36%). In all but one trial[24] the percentage of subjects reporting side effects was higher in the antibiotic arm; subsequent pooling of data showed that a course of antibiotic was associated with a non-significant increase in the risk of side effects from antibiotic (relative risk 1.51 (0.86 to 2.64)) (fig 4). When the one trial which reported an increase in side effects from placebo was excluded,[24] the heterogeneity between trials was reduced and side effects were significantly associated with antibiotic use (relative risk 1.9 (1.19 to 3.02), χ^2 test for heterogeneity = 1.73, df = 4, P > 0.5).

BMJ VOLUME 316   21 MARCH 1998

Discussion

This systematic review shows that antibiotic treatment has no effect on the resolution of acute cough. For both measures of efficacy—the proportion of subjects coughing and the proportion whose symptoms had not improved at days 7-11—antibiotic was no different from placebo. Furthermore, treatment with antibiotic may incur side effects in a few patients.

Shortcomings

This review has several shortcomings. Firstly, the outcomes chosen and assessed in each of the randomised trials were varied and different. Consequently, when the results were pooled several important outcomes were reported only in some of the trials and were measured in different ways. For example, time off work was measured as a continuous outcome in two trials,[23 28] as a categorical outcome in three others,[21 22 25] as a categorical and continuous outcome in one trial,[27] and not at all in the remaining trials (M Stephenson, unpublished data).[24 26]

Secondly, more recent generic scores for measuring the quality of life were not used in any of the trials, once again limiting the propensity to combine the results. Therefore important information for patients such as the effect of antibiotic on quality of life and on return to work is not reported.

Finally, the timing of assessment differed between trials. Such differences make it difficult to measure the clinical course of acute cough. These shortcomings reflect the difficulty in combining results from pragmatic randomised trials that examine outcomes based on illness in general practice. Nevertheless, substantially important differences between antibiotic and placebo are unlikely to be present in these other outcomes: individual trials did not report any substantial benefit of antibiotic in the outcomes that we did not consider in this systematic review.

Diagnosis and prognosis

The clinical course of resolution of acute cough was different between trials (fig 1). Such differences reflect the fact that acute cough is primarily diagnosed on history and examination alone. Additional diagnostic tests such as sputum culture and chest radiography are seldom used in general practice,[1 9 12] so diagnostic classification is imprecise. The diagnostic nomenclature has also changed over time. For example, an early non-randomised study of acute respiratory infection[38] found that the signs reported by the enrolled cohort were no different from those in subjects classed as having acute bronchitis in the 1980s.[22-25 27] In addition, the relation between diagnostic category and likelihood of bacterial infection is poorly defined and uncertain in clinical practice.

Inevitably, the diagnostic heterogeneity in each of the randomised controlled trials has been reflected in differences in the reported resolution of cough or illness (fig 1). Results from cohort studies suggest that it may take up to three or four weeks before cough has resolved and general wellbeing returned in patients with acute bronchitis.[39]

Implications

In the clinical context of everyday management of acute cough in general practice, treatment with antibiotics is common. The variation in rate of prescribing antibiotics varies substantially between countries. One fifth of consultations in the Netherlands end with an antibiotic being prescribed, up to 80% in the United Kingdom, and an even higher proportion in the United States.[40-42] Results from our systematic review suggest that most patients receive no benefit from antibiotic treatment.

We calculated the number needed to treat (11) and the number needed to harm (15) if we accepted that the outcome of proportion of subjects who reported clinical improvement was balanced with the proportion likely to have side effects from taking antibiotic. For every 100 people treated with antibiotic, nine would report an improvement after 7-11 days if they revisited their general practitioner but at the expense of seven others who would have side effects from the antibiotic. The resolution of illness in the remaining 84 people would not be affected by treatment with antibiotic.

One of the higher quality trials reported that the prognostic factors of frequent cough combined with feeling ill at entry were associated with beneficial effects from antibiotic treatment.[26] The same trial also reported that people aged over 55 derived benefit from such treatment.[26] These findings are consistent with the greater prevalence of bacterial infection and subsequent infection of the lower respiratory tract in people aged over 55 and increased rates of hospital admission of elderly people.[7 10 43] However, until prospective randomised controlled trials test whether age, feeling unwell, and frequent cough predict a poor clinical outcome or bacterial infection and also influence clinical

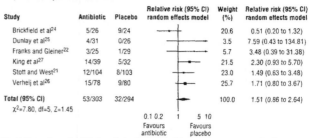

Proportion of subjects with side effects

Study	Antibiotic	Placebo	Relative risk (95% CI) random effects model	Weight (%)	Relative risk (95% CI) random effects model
Brickfield et al[24]	5/26	9/24		20.6	0.51 (0.20 to 1.32)
Dunlay et al[25]	4/31	0/26		3.5	7.59 (0.43 to 134.81)
Franks and Gleiner[22]	3/25	1/29		5.7	3.48 (0.39 to 31.38)
King et al[27]	14/39	5/32		21.5	2.30 (0.93 to 5.70)
Stott and West[21]	12/104	8/103		23.0	1.49 (0.63 to 3.48)
Verheij et al[26]	15/78	9/80		25.7	1.71 (0.80 to 3.67)
Total (95% CI)	53/303	32/294		100.0	1.51 (0.86 to 2.64)

$\chi^2 = 7.80$, df=5, Z=1.45

0.1 0.2   1   5 10
Favours antibiotic   Favours placebo

Fig 4 Comparison of antibiotic and placebo treatment on rate of reporting of side effects

---

Key messages

- Acute cough, with or without sputum, is a common reason for consulting a general practitioner

- Although antibiotic treatment is common for this condition, its likely benefits and side effects have not been measured

- This systematic review reports the outcome of nine randomised controlled trials that compared antibiotic with placebo in patients with acute cough

- Resolution of cough and clinical improvement at follow up was no different in the two groups

- The benefits of antibiotic treatment seem to be marginal for most patients with acute cough and may be outweighed by the side effects of treatment and quality of life outcomes associated with antibiotic treatment, treatment based on these prognostic variables will remain speculative.

Apart from the side effects of treatment, three other factors need to be considered by a clinician before prescribing antibiotics. Firstly, the cost of prescribing antibiotic is important. A recent decision analysis suggests that the most cost effective strategy is to withold antibiotic and treat only patients with persistent cough.[44] Secondly, treatment with antibiotic may change patients' expectations about future episodes of acute cough. Observational research suggests that patients' expectations may increase and influence subsequent workload among general practitioners.[41][45] A recently published open randomised trial of antibiotic for sore throat showed that patients prescribed antibiotic were more likely to consult in the future than were those whose symptoms were treated.[46] Qualitative research suggests that patients' satisfaction is likely to be higher when their expectations are addressed than when antibiotic is prescribed.[17] Finally, bacterial resistance to antibiotics is becoming increasingly common.[48] A liberal prescribing policy by general practitioners managing acute bronchitis is likely to make this situation worse.

Conclusions

This systematic review shows that antibiotic is unlikely to alter the course of illness in most adult patients presenting with acute cough. A minority may have side effects from treatment. When managing individual patients the potential risks from treatment—including side effects, costs of antibiotic, alteration in consulting behaviour, and increased bacterial resistance—should all be considered before initiating treatment.

We thank the following for providing extra data, clarifying data from published studies, or providing information about unpublished studies: Chris van Weel, Peter Franks, John Howie, Laurent Kaiser, Dana King, Amy Schende, Mike Stephenson, Siewert Thomas, Nigel Stott, Murray Tilyard, and Theo Verheij. We also thank the following for comments on the manuscript: Mike Crilly, Jon Deeks, Tim Lancaster, Debbie Sharp, and Michael Whitfield. Finally, we would particularly like to thank Debbie Jones for help with the searching and Matthias Egger for helping us with methodological dilemmas.

Contributors: TF formulated the research question, spoke to authors of randomised controlled trials, extracted and analysed data, and wrote the first draft of the manuscript. NS extracted data, spoke to authors of randomised controlled trials, and contributed to writing the manuscript. TT searched for randomised controlled trials and contacted authors for unpublished studies. TF is the guarantor for the paper.

Funding: The Royal College of General Practitioners Scientific Foundation Board.

Conflict of interest: None.

1 Verheij T, Kaptein A, Mulder J. Acute bronchitis: aetiology, symptoms and treatment. Fam Pract 1989;6:66-9.
2 Gwaltney JM. Acute bronchitis. In: Mandell GL, Bennet JE, Dolin R, eds. Principles and practice of infectious diseases. 4th ed. New York: Churchill Livingstone, 1995:606-8.
3 World Organisation of National Colleges and Academies of General Practice. An international classification of health problems in primary health care (ICHPPC-2). 3rd ed. Oxford: Oxford University Press, 1983.
4 Boldy DA, Skidmore SJ, Ayres JG. Acute bronchitis in the community: clinical features, infective factors, changes in pulmonary function and bronchial reactivity to histamine. Respir Med 1990;84:377-85.
5 Royal College of General Practitioners, Office of Population Censuses and Surveys, Department of Health. Morbidity statistics from general practice. Fourth national study, 1991-1992. London: HMSO, 1995.
6 MRC Working Party on Acute Respiratory Virus Infections. A collaborative study of the aetiology of acute respiratory infections in Britain, 1961-4. BMJ 1965;ii:319-26.
7 Garibaldi RA. Epidemiology of community-acquired respiratory tract infections in adults. Am J Med 1985;78:32-7.
8 King DE, Muncie HL. High prevalence of Mycoplasma pneumoniae in patients with respiratory tract symptoms: a rapid detection method. J Fam Pract 1991;32:529-31.
9 Johnson PH, MacFarlane JT, Humphreys H. How is sputum microbiology used in general practice? Respir Med 1996;90:87-8.
10 Macfarlane J, Colville A, Guion A, Macfarlane R, Rose D. Prospective study of aetiology and outcome of adult lower-respiratory-tract infections in the community. Lancet 1993;341:511-4.
11 Örtqvist A. Respiratory infection: community acquired respiratory infection. Lancet 1993;341:529-30.
12 Verheij T, Hermans J, Kaptein A, Wijkel D, Mulder J. Acute bronchitis: general practitioners' views regarding diagnosis and treatment. Fam Pract 1990;7:175-80.
13 Howie JR, Richardson IM, Gill G, Durno D. Respiratory illness and antibiotic use in general practice. J R Coll Gen Pract 1971;21:657-63.
14 Antibiotics and respiratory illness [editorial]. BMJ 1974;ii:1.
15 Wyatt T, Passmore C, Morrow N, Reilly P. Antibiotic prescribing: the need for a policy in general practice. BMJ 1990;300:441-4.
16 Orr P, Scherer K, Macdonald A, Moffatt M. Randomised placebo-controlled trials of antibiotics for acute bronchitis: a critical review of the literature. J Fam Pract 1993;36:507-12.
17 MacKay DN. Treatment of acute bronchitis in adults without underlying lung disease. J Gen Intern Med 1996;11:557-62.
18 Gonzales R, Sande M. What will it take to stop physicians from prescribing antibiotics in acute bronchitis? Lancet 1995;345:665-6.
19 Wise R. Antibiotics for the uncommon cold. Lancet 1996;347:1499.
20 Howie J, Clark G. Double-blind trial of early demethylchlortetracycline in minor respiratory illness in general practice. Lancet 1970;ii:1099-102.
21 Stott N, West R. Randomised controlled trial of antibiotics in patients with cough and purulent sputum. BMJ 1976;ii:556-9.
22 Franks P, Gleiner J. The treatment of acute bronchitis with trimethoprim and sulfamethoxazole. J Fam Pract 1984;19:185-90.
23 Williamson H. A randomised, controlled trial of doxycycline in the treatment of acute bronchitis. J Fam Pract 1984;19:481-6.
24 Brickfield F, Carter W, Johnson R. Erythromycin in the treatment of acute bronchitis in a community practice. J Fam Pract 1986;23:119-22.
25 Dunlay J, Reinhardt R, Donn L. A placebo-controlled, double blind trial of erythromycin in adults with acute bronchitis. J Fam Pract 1987;25:137-41.
26 Verheij T, Hermans J, Mulder J. Effects of doxycycline in patients with acute cough and purulent sputum: a double blind placebo controlled trial. Br J Gen Pract 1994;44:400-4.
27 King D, Williams CW, Bishop L, Shechter A. Effectiveness of erythromycin in the treatment of acute bronchitis. J Fam Pract 1996;42:601-5.
28 Scherl E, Riegler S, Cooper J. Doxycycline in acute bronchitis: a randomized double-blind trial. Journal of the Kentucky Medical Association 1987;85:539-41.
29 Dickerson K, Scherer R, Lefebvre C. Identifying relevant studies for systematic reviews. In: Chalmers I, Altman D, eds. Systematic reviews. London: BMJ Publishing Group, 1995:17-36.
30 Cochrane Collaboration. The Cochrane Library. Issue 2 ed. Oxford: Update Software, 1997.
31 Mulrow CD, Oxman AD. Cochrane Collaboration Handbook (updated 9 December 1996). In: The Cochrane Collaboration. ed. The Cochrane Library (database on disc and CDROM). Issue 2 ed. Oxford: Update Software, 1996.
32 Hennekens C, Buring J. Epidemiology in medicine. Boston: Little, Brown, 1987.
33 L'Abbe KA, Detsky AS. O'Rourke K. Meta-analysis in clinical research. Ann Intern Med 1987;107:224-33.
34 Petitti DB. Meta-analysis, decision analysis and cost-effectiveness analysis. Methods for quantitative synthesis in medicine. New York: Oxford University Press, 1994.
35 Sackett D, Richardson WS, Rosenberg W, Haynes RB. Evidence-based medicine: how to practise and teach EBM. London: Churchill Livingstone, 1996.
36 Thomas S. Antibiotics for cough and purulent sputum. BMJ 1978;ii:1374.
37 Kaiser L, Lew D, Hirschel B, Auckenthaler R, Morabia A, Heald A, et al. Effects of antibiotic treatment in the subset of common-cold patients who have bacteria in nasopharyngeal secretions. Lancet 1996;347:1507-10.
38 Jones PH, Bigham R, Manning PR. Use of antibiotics in nonbacterial respiratory infections. JAMA 1953;99:262-4.
39 Verheij T, Hermans J, Kaptein A, Mulder J. Acute bronchitis: course of symptoms and restrictions in patients daily activities. Scand J Primary Health Care 1995;13:8-12.
40 Kuyvenhoven M, de Melker R, Van der Velden K. Prescription of antibiotics and prescribers' characteristics. A study into prescription of antibiotics in upper respiratory tract infections in general practice. Fam Pract 1993;10:366-70.
41 Davey P, Rutherford D, Graham B, Lynch B, Malek M. Repeat consultations after antibiotic prescribing for respiratory infections: a study in one general practice. Br J Gen Pract 1994;44:509-13.
42 Mainous AG, Hueston W, Clark JR. Antibiotics and upper respiratory infection. J Fam Pract 1996;42:357-61.
43 Verheij T. Antibiotics in acute bronchitis. Lancet 1995;345:1244.
44 Hueston WJ. Antibiotics: neither cost effective nor "cough" effective. J Fam Pract 1997;44:261-5.
45 Howie JGR, Hutchison KR. Antibiotics and respiratory illness in general practice: prescribing policy and work load. BMJ 1978;ii:1342.
46 Little P, Gould C, Williamson I, Warner G, Gantley M, Kinmonth AL. Reattendance and complications in a randomised trial of prescribing strategies for sore throat: the medicalising effect of prescribing antibiotics. BMJ 1997;315:350-2.
47 Hamm RM, Hicks RJ, Bemben DA. Antibiotics and respiratory infections: are patients more satisfied when expectations are met? J Fam Pract 1996;43:56-62.
48 Verkatesun P, Innes JA. Antibiotic resistance in common acute respiratory pathogens. Thorax 1995;50:481-3.

(Accepted 18 November 1997)

Citation:

Are the results of this systematic review of therapy valid?

Is it a systematic review of randomised trials of the treatment you're interested in?

Does it include a methods section that describes:
• finding and including all the relevant trials?
• assessing their individual validity?

Were the results consistent from study to study?

Are the valid results of this systematic review important?

Is there a statistically significant benefit of treatment?

Do the confidence intervals confirm or exclude clinically significant benefit or harm?

Can you apply this valid, important evidence from a systematic review in caring for your patient?

Do these results apply to your patient?

Is your patient so different from those in the
systematic review that its results can't help you?

How great would the potential benefit of therapy actually be for your individual patient?

Many meta-analyses report their results as odds ratios.
There is a table available for calculating the NNT from
odds ratios and the patient's expected event rate
(PEER) (see p. 141 of *Evidence-based Medicine*).

In this case, however, the authors have used relative
risk, which can be more simply applied to the PEER.
The expected benefits of treatment can be obtained
by multiplying the PEER by the relative risk reduction
(1-RR). This yields the ARR. The NNT is 1/ARR.

Are your patient's values and preferences satisfied by the regimen and its consequences?

Do your patient and you have a clear assessment of
their values and preferences?

Are they met by this regimen and its consequences?

Does the review suggest differences in the efficacy of therapy in some subgroups of patients? If so, should you believe apparent qualitative differences in the efficacy of therapy in these subgroups? Only if you can say 'yes' to all of the following:

Do they really make biologic and clinical sense?

Is the qualitative difference both clinically (beneficial
for some but useless or harmful for others) and
statistically significant?

Was this difference hypothesised before the study
began (rather than the product of dredging the
data), and has it been confirmed in other,
independent studies?

Was this one of just a few subgroup analyses
carried out in this study?

Additional notes

Citation: Fahey T, Stocks N, Thomas T (1998) Quantitative systematic review of randomised controlled trials comparing antibiotics with placebo for acute cough in adults. *BMJ.* 316: 906–10

Are the results of this systematic review of therapy valid?

Is it a systematic review of randomised trials of the treatment you're interested in?	**Yes, although it does not include children, which is a group in whom you are interested.**
Does it include a methods section that describes: • finding and including all the relevant trials? • assessing their individual validity?	**Yes.** **Yes, trials were scored on four criteria: selection bias, performance bias, attrition bias and detection bias.**
Were the results consistent from study to study?	**There was some heterogeneity in reporting of results. However, trials which reported similar outcomes showed consistent results for reported resolution of illness.**

Are the valid results of this systematic review important?

Is there a statistically significant benefit of treatment?	**No. The meta-analysis does not show a statistically significant effect of antibiotics on proportion of patients with cough at follow-up, or on the proportion of patients who had not improved clinically at follow-up.**
Do the confidence intervals confirm or exclude clinically significant benefit or harm?	**Although the effect is not significant (the confidence intervals include 1), the estimates for the relative risk reduction are in the direction of benefit from treatment. The lower bounds of the confidence intervals include relative risks of 0.73 for cough, and 0.36 for clinical improvement.**

Can you apply this valid, important evidence from a systematic review in caring for your patients?

Do these results apply to your patients?

Is your patient so different from those in the systematic review that its results can't help you?	In drawing up a practice policy, it is important to know whether there are some patients who will benefit from antibiotics. On the basis of one trial, the authors suggest that patients over the age of 55, who were ill at entry to the trial, might be a group who benefit from antibiotics.

How great would the potential benefit of therapy actually be for your patients?

Many meta-analyses report their results as odds ratios. There is a table available for calculating the NNT from odds ratios and the patient's expected event rate (PEER) (See p. 141 of *Evidence-based Medicine*). In this case, however, the authors have used relative risk, which can be more simply applied to the PEER. The expected benefits of treatment can be obtained by multiplying the PEER by the relative risk reduction (1-RR). This yields the ARR. The NNT is 1/ARR.	For cough at follow-up, the risk in the control group is about 40%. The ARR = 0.4 x (1 – 0.85) = 0.06. The NNT is 1/0.06 = 16 (95% CI 9 to infinity). For clinical improvement, the risk in the control group is 24%. The ARR = 0.24 – (1 – 0.62) = 0.09. The NNT = 1/0.09 = 11 (95% CI 6 to infinity). For side-effects, the risk in the placebo group is about 11%. The absolute risk increase is (0.11 x 1.51) – 0.11 = 0.06. NNH = 1/0.06 = 16

Are your patient's values and preferences satisfied by the regimen and its consequences?

Do your patient and you have a clear assessment of their values and preferences?	Needs to be assessed in each patient: when they understand the size of the possible benefit, and the risk of side-effects, some patients may not wish to take an antibiotic.
Are they met by this regimen and its consequences?	Needs to be assessed in each patient.

Does the review suggest differences in the efficacy of therapy in some subgroups of patients? If so, should you believe apparent qualitative differences in the efficacy of therapy in these subgroups? Only if you can say 'yes' to all of the following:

Do they really make biologic and clinical sense?
In this example, no formal sub-group analyses were performed. However, the authors do note, with caution, that one study suggested benefit in older patients who were more ill at entry to the study.

Is the qualitative difference both clinically (beneficial for some but useless or harmful for others) and statistically significant?

Was this difference hypothesised before the study began (rather than the product of dredging the data), and has it been confirmed in other, independent studies?

Was this one of just a few subgroup analyses carried out in this study?

Additional notes

Clinical Bottom Line

For patients presenting with acute cough in general practice (excluding patients with chronic obstructive airways disease), there is no statistically significant benefit from antibiotics.

Citation

Fahey T, Stocks N, Thomas T (1998) Quantitative systematic review of randomised controlled trials comparing antibiotics with placebo for acute cough in adults. *BMJ*. **316:** 906–10.

Clinical Question

In patients presenting with acute cough in general practice, do antibiotics lead to reduction in symptoms (and/or increase in side-effects) compared to symptomatic treatments alone?

Search Terms

MEDLINE search using terms 'cough' and 'antibiotic' and 'systematic review'.

The Study

Systematic review and meta-analysis of nine randomised controlled trials that compared antibiotic with placebo in patients (age >12 years) presenting with acute cough/respiratory infection in the community. Patients with chronic obstructive airways disease were not included.

There was variation in how respiratory infection was defined in the different studies, and in the outcomes reported. In this review, the authors concentrate on three outcomes: proportion of subjects with productive cough at 7–11 days; proportion of subjects who had not improved at 7–11 days; and proportion of subjects reporting side-effects from taking antibiotic or placebo.

The Evidence

1   No statistically significant benefit of antibiotic for resolution of cough at days 7–11 (relative risk 0.85, 95% CI 0.73 to 1.00), NNT 16 (95% CI 9 to infinity).

2   No statistically significant benefit of antibiotic for clinical improvement at days 7–11 (relative risk 0.62, 95% CI 0.36 to 1.09), NNT 11 (95% CI 6 to infinity).

3   Antibiotics were associated with a non-significant increase in the risk of side-effects from antibiotic (relative risk 1.51, 0.86 to 2.64), NNH 16.

Comments

1   Although not statistically significant, the confidence intervals around the estimates do not exclude a potentially useful clinical benefit. However, this will have to be balanced against risk of side-effects. The authors estimate that for every 100 patients treated with antibiotic, nine would report an improvement after 7–11 days but at the expense of seven who would suffer side-effects.

2   One well conducted study suggested that patients who were feeling very ill at entry and/or were aged over 55, derived benefit from antibiotics. This may be a group in whom bacterial infection is more common, where it may be reasonable to use antibiotics.

CAT – ANTIBIOTICS FOR ACUTE COUGH IN GENERAL PRACTICE

Appraised by Tim Lancaster.
Expiry date: January 2000.

PART A
Presentations
(comfortably 3 per hour)

1 In groups of 10 or less, participants will present their critical appraisals they have carried out on clinical topics of their choice.

2 Reports will state the three-part clinical question, summarise the search in one sentence, critically appraise the best article found, and discuss how the appraisal was integrated with clinical expertise and applied on that (or a similar, subsequent) patient.

3 A total of 15 minutes will be allotted for each presentation: 10 minutes for presentation and 5 minutes for group discussion.

PART B
Searching for evidence on the WWW

We will show you how to access the web and introduce you to the web page for the Centre for Evidence-based Medicine in Oxford (http://cebm.jr2.ox.ac.uk/), where there are data banks of clinically useful measures on the precision and accuracy of clinical exam and lab test results (SpPins, SnNouts, sensitivities, specificities, likelihood ratios), the power of prognostic factors and therapy (NNTs, RRRs and the like), plus the CATMaker and links to several other centres and sources of evidence.

NOTES ON THE INTERNET

The Internet: why bother?

- Networking with colleagues.
- Getting hold of useful documents for free.
- Publishing useful information for free.
- Bypassing traditional publishers and online vendors.

EBM on the Internet

- e-mail discussion list (run by Mailbase):
  evidence-based-health@mailbase.ac.uk

To join send an e-mail to **mailbase@mailbase.ac.uk** with an empty subject field and the following as the only text of the message itself: **join evidence-based-health Joe Bloggs**

To get list of mailbase discussion lists, send this command in the same way to the same address: **find lists medical**

To get a mailbase user guide, send the command: **send mailbase user-guide**

- The EBM Toolbox (the CEBM World-Wide Web site)
  http://cebm.jr2.ox.ac.uk/

See links to other sites (especially SCHARR) in Other Resources. It also has:

- a glossary of EBHC terms and research methodologies
- how to focus a clinical question
- educational prescriptions
- hints on how to optimise MEDLINE searches
- detailed definitions and examples of NNTs, SpPins and SnNouts, likelihood ratios, pre-test probabilities, prognostic indicators
- scenarios used in the teaching packs at our workshops
- worksheets for critical appraisal

Searching for stuff on the Web

- Use other people's links to good sites. An excellent place to start for this is the Netting the Evidence and SCHARR Project at Sheffield: **http://www.shef.ac.uk/~scharr/ir/netting.html**
- To find your own good sites, use the search engines, such as:

Altavista:	**www.altavista.com**
Excite:	**www.excite.com**
Lycos:	**www.lycos.com**
Yahoo!:	**www.yahoo.com**

There is a good site with links to all the best internet search engines at: **http://alt.venus.co.uk/weed/search/welcome.htm**

- The browser's **Find** button can help to scan large pages
- Use **Bookmarks** to record good sites
- You can search MEDLINE on the Internet at various sites, including PubMed: **http://www3.ncbi.nlm.nih.gov/PubMed/**

TCP/IP (Transmission Control Protocol / Internet Protocol): the lingua franca, a common language of protocols which allows different computers to exchange information.

- It is a loose association of networks of computers which has generated a massive publishing and communications arena.

- Every computer on the Internet (host) has its own unique IP address which defines where it is and enables other computers to send and forward messages to it. There is no central server for the Internet, so it is both robust (nearly impossible to destroy) and chaotic (nearly impossible to control).

- Typically, you will use your computer to log in to a host which has an Internet connection and which has an account for your use. If you are lucky, your machine will be a host in itself, which means others can log in to your machine and use it (for example, see Telnet).

- You will use the Internet from a particular domain (locality) which will have local management of services.

- the set of five services which are supported by the Internet protocols are:

E-mail (SMTP)	Text messages sent to a person: **user@host.domain**	User decides when to read, one to many with mailing lists, e.g. mailbase.	Not 100% reliable; Internet e-mail not universal in NHS; addresses can be obscure.
USENET News Groups (NNTP)	USENET servers contain textual discussion lists where users add their comments to a discussion.	Thousands of topics to choose from; can be a good source of advice.	Difficult to find relevant group; can be a source of abuse!
Telnet	Allows you to connect to a host computer across the Internet and use it as if you were sitting in front of it.	Allows you to use the resources of the host computer.	Usually just text-based commands, i.e. no Windows; you need an account with the host to be able to do this.
File transfer protocol (FTP)	You can log on to a host, browse its directories and exchange files efficiently (including programs).	You don't need authorisation (anonymous FTP means you type 'Guest' as a login name and your e-mail address as password).	Can be very difficult to browse effectively (you have to know where to look and download to see what you are getting).
WWW (http)	Use a browser program to read multimedia documents (and programs) stored on any Internet host running the http program.	Instant publishing. Login, addressing and downloading with one click of the mouse. Can be searched and marked.	Imagine the Bodleian with all the books shuffled and dumped on the floor.

Usually, different services will be managed locally by a specific host (a server) which may or may not be the same machine.

Reference
Krol E (1994) The Whole Internet: users' guide and catalogue. O'Reilly.

PART A — Presentations

The other half of the participants will present their patients, questions, critically appraised topics, and clinical conclusions.

PART B — Feedback and celebration

The final portion of the session (and course!) can be spent evaluating the course. The first of the attached forms (**Evaluation of 'practising EBM'**) permits written feedback about this course, and a discussion will be held on the general issues within it.

The second form (**'Am I practising EBM?'**) is a checklist that you may want to apply to your own performance in order to determine whether you are beginning to apply the self-directed, problem-based learning and EBM skills in your own practice and in your clinical teaching.

Special attention will be given to discussing and deciding what to do with what has been learned, and how to continue to improve and use this set of clinical, EBM and self-directed learning skills.

EVALUATION OF 'PRACTISING EBM'

Please rate the items using the following scale from 1 to 5 where:

1 – awful   3 – adequate   5 – excellent

1   *How well were your objectives met in this course?*

   a Learning how to ask answerable clinical questions related to pts you care for on the clinical service

                                      1   2   3   4   5

   b Learning how to search for the best evidence

                                        1   2   3   4   5

   c Learning how to critically appraise the medical literature

                                        1   2   3   4   5

   d Learning how to integrate this literature with your clinical expertise and to apply the results in your clinical practice

                                        1   2   3   4   5

   e Learning how to evaluate your performance

                                        1   2   3   4   5

2   *Therapy Session*

		1	2	3	4	5
a	Relevance of the session	1	2	3	4	5
b	Appropriateness of the article	1	2	3	4	5
c	Organisation of the session	1	2	3	4	5
d	Teaching during the session	1	2	3	4	5

3   *Diagnosis Session*

a	Relevance of the session	1	2	3	4	5
b	Appropriateness of the article	1	2	3	4	5
c	Organisation of the session	1	2	3	4	5
d	Teaching during the session	1	2	3	4	5

3   *Prognosis Session*

a	Relevance of the session	1	2	3	4	5
b	Appropriateness of the article	1	2	3	4	5
c	Organisation of the session	1	2	3	4	5
d	Teaching during the session	1	2	3	4	5

4   *Systematic Review Session*

a	Relevance of the session	1	2	3	4	5
b	Appropriateness of the article	1	2	3	4	5
c	Organisation of the session	1	2	3	4	5
d	Teaching during the session	1	2	3	4	5

Session 7 – Presentations, feedback & celebration

5 *Harm Session*

   a Relevance of the session   1   2   3   4   5

   b Appropriateness of the article 1   2   3   4   5

   c Organisation of the session   1   2   3   4   5

   d Teaching during the session   1   2   3   4   5

6 *Final Presentation Sessions*

   a Relevance of the presentations 1   2   3   4   5

   b Quality of the presentations   1   2   3   4   5

   c Quality of the discussions   1   2   3   4   5

   d Organisation of the session   1   2   3   4   5

7 *How well do you think this course will help you prepare for your Membership Exams?*

                                           1   2   3   4   5

8 *Overall rating of the course*

                                         1   2   3   4   5

9 *What was the best thing about this course (that should be preserved and expanded in future courses)?*

10 *What was the worst thing about this course (that should be removed from future courses of this sort)?*

11 *Other comments and suggestions:*

Many thanks

AM I PRACTISING EBM?

A self-evaluation in asking answerable questions.

a   Are you asking any questions at all?

b   Are you:
  • using the guides to asking 3-part questions?
  • using educational prescriptions
  • asking your colleagues: 'What's your evidence for that?'

c   Is your success rate of asking answerable questions rising?

d   How do your questions compare with those of respected colleagues?

A self-evaluation in finding the best external evidence.

a   Are you searching at all?

b   Do you know the best sources of current evidence for your clinical discipline?

c   Have you achieved immediate access to searching hardware, software and the best evidence for your clinical discipline?

d   Are you finding useful external evidence from a widening array of sources?

e   Are you becoming more efficient in your searching?

f   Are you using MeSH headings, thesaurus, limiters, and intelligent free text when searching MEDLINE?

g   How do your searches compare with those of research librarians or other respected colleagues who have a passion for providing best current patient care?

A self-evaluation in critically appraising the evidence for its validity and potential usefulness.

a   Are you critically appraising external evidence at all?

b   Are the critical appraisal guides becoming easier to apply?

c   Are you becoming more accurate and efficient in applying some of the critical appraisal measures (such as likelihood ratios, NNTs and the like)?

d   Are you creating any CATs?

e   Are you using the CATMaker?

f   Have you shared any of the CATs you've made with your colleagues or other learners?

A self-evaluation in integrating the critical appraisal with your clinical expertise and applying the result in your clinical practice.

a   Are you integrating your critical appraisals into your practice at all?

b   Are you becoming more accurate and efficient in adjusting some of the critical appraisal measures to fit your individual patients (pre-test probabilities, NNT/f, etc.)?

c   Can you explain (and resolve) disagreements about management decisions in terms of this integration?

d   Have you conducted any clinical decision analyses?

e   Have you carried out any audits of your diagnostic, therapeutic, or other EBM performance?

Session 7 – Presentations, feedback & celebration

A self-evaluation in teaching EBM.

a   When did you last issue an educational prescription?

b   Are you helping your trainees learn how to ask answerable (3-part) questions?

c   Are you teaching and modelling searching skills (or making sure that your trainees learn them)?

d   Are you teaching and modelling critical appraisal skills?

e   Are you teaching and modelling the generation of CATs?

f   Are you teaching and modelling the integration of best evidence with individual clinical expertise?

g   Are you developing new ways of evaluating the effectiveness of your teaching?[1]

h   Are you developing new EBM educational materials?[2]

A self-evaluation of your own continuing professional development.

a   Are you a member of an EBM-style journal club?

b   Have you participated in or tutored at one of the workshops on how to practice or teach EBM?

c   Have you joined the evidence-based-health e-mail discussion group?

d   Have you established links with other practitioners or teachers of EBM?

[1] If so, please share them with the developers of this course!

[2] If so, please add them to the bank of EBM educational resources that the Oxford Centre for Evidence-based Medicine shares with other educators around the world.

Glossary of terms you are likely to encounter in your clinical reading

This glossary is intended to provide guidance as to the meanings of terms you will come across frequently in clinical articles, especially when they appear in EBM journals.

Absolute risk reduction (ARR) – see *Treatment effects*

Case-control study – a study which involves identifying patients who have the outcome of interest (cases) and control patients without the same outcome, and looking back to see if they had the exposure of interest (*see also Review of study designs*).

Case-series – a report on a series of patients with an outcome of interest. No control group is involved.

Clinical practice guideline – is a systematically developed statement designed to assist practitioner and patient decisions about appropriate health care for specific clinical circumstances.

Cohort study – involves identification of two groups (cohorts) of patients, one which did receive the exposure of interest, and one which did not, and following these cohorts forward for the outcome of interest (*see also Review of study designs*).

Confidence interval (CI) – the range within which we would expect the true value of a statistical measure to lie. The CI is usually accompanied by a percentage value which shows the level of confidence that the true value lies within this range. For example, for an NNT of 10 with a 95% CI of 5 to 15, we would have 95% confidence that the true NNT value was between 5 and 15.

Control event rate (CER) – see *Treatment effects*.

Cost-benefit analysis – assesses whether the cost of an intervention is worth the benefit by measuring both in the same units; monetary units are usually used.

Cost-effectiveness analysis – measures the net cost of providing a service as well as the outcomes obtained. Outcomes are reported in a single unit of measurement.

Cost-utility analysis – converts effects into personal preferences (or utilities) and describes how much it costs for some additional quality gain (e.g. cost per additional quality-adjusted life-year, or QALY).

Crossover study design – the administration of two or more experimental therapies one after the other in a specified or random order to the same group of patients (*see also Review of study designs*).

Cross-sectional study – the observation of a defined population at a single point in time or time interval. Exposure and outcome are determined simultaneously (*see also Review of study designs*).

Decision analysis – is the application of explicit, quantitative methods that quantify prognoses, treatment effects, and patient values in order to analyse a decision under conditions of uncertainty.

Ecological survey – a survey based on aggregated data for some population as it exists at some point or points in time; to investigate the relationship of an exposure to a known or presumed risk factor for a specified outcome.

Event rate – the proportion of patients in a group in whom the event is observed. Thus, if out of 100 patients, the event is observed in 27, the event rate is 0.27. Control event rate (CER) and experimental event rate (EER) are used to refer to this in control and experimental groups of patients respectively. The patient expected event rate (PEER) refers to the rate of events we'd expect in a patient who received no treatment or conventional treatment – *see **Treatment effects***.

Evidence-based health care – extends the application of the principles of evidence-based medicine (*see* below) to all professions associated with health care, including purchasing and management.

Evidence-based medicine – the conscientious, explicit and judicious use of current best evidence in making decisions about the care of individual patients. The practice of evidence-based medicine means integrating individual clinical expertise with the best available external clinical evidence from systematic research. *See also* Sackett *et al.* (1996) EBM: What it is and what it isn't. *BMJ* **312:** 71–2.

Experimental event rate (EER) – *see **Treatment effects***.

Likelihood ratio (LR) – the likelihood that a given test result would be expected in a patient with the target disorder compared to the likelihood that that same result would be expected in a patient without the target disorder.

Calculation of sensitivity/specificity/LR:

	DISEASE POSITIVE	DISEASE NEGATIVE
TEST POSITIVE	a	b
TEST NEGATIVE	c	d

Sensitivity = $a/(a+c)$

$$LR+ = \frac{\text{sensitivity}}{1-\text{specificity}} = \frac{a/(a+c)}{b/(b+d)}$$

Specificity = $d/(b+d)$

$$LR- = \frac{(1-\text{sensitivity})}{\text{specificity}} = \frac{c/(a+c)}{d/(b+d)}$$

Positive predictive value = $a/(a+b)$ Negative predictive value = $d/(c+d)$

Meta-analysis – is an overview that uses quantitative methods to summarise the results.

N-of-1 trials – in such trials, the patient undergoes pairs of treatment periods organised so that one period involves the use of the experimental treatment and one period involves the use of an alternate or placebo therapy. The patients and physician are blinded, if possible, and outcomes are monitored. Treatment periods are replicated until the clinician and patient are convinced that the treatments are definitely different or definitely not different.

Negative predictive value – proportion of people with a negative test who are free of the target disorder (*see also **Likelihood ratio***).

Number needed to treat (NNT) – is the inverse of the absolute risk reduction and is the number of patients that need to be treated to prevent one bad outcome – *see **Treatment effects***.

Odds – a ratio of non-events to events. If the event rate for a disease is 0.1 (10%), its non-event rate is 0.9 and therefore its odds are 9:1. Note that this is not the same expression as the inverse of event rate.

Odds ratio (OR) – is the odds of having the target disorder in the experimental group relative to the odds in favour of having the target disorder in the control group (in prospective case-control studies, overviews) or the odds in favour of being exposed in subjects with the target disorder divided by the odds in favour of being exposed in control subjects (without the target disorder).

Calculations of OR/RR for use of trimethoprim-sulfamethoxazole prophylaxis in cirrhosis:

	Adverse event occurs (infectious complication)	Adverse event does not occur (no infectious complication)	Totals
Exposed to treatment (experimental)	1	29	30
	a	b	a+b
Not exposed to treatment (control)	c	d	c+d
	9	21	30
Totals	a+c	b+d	a+b+c+d
	10	50	60

CER = $c/(c+d)$ = 0.30
EER = $a/(a+b)$ = 0.033
Control Event Odds = c/d = 0.43
Experimental Event Odds = a/b = 0.034
Relative Risk = EER/CER = 0.11
Relative Odds = Odds Ratio = $(a/b)/(c/d)$ = ad/bc = 0.08

Patient expected event rate – *see* **Treatment effects**.

Overview – is a systematic review and summary of the medical literature (*see* **meta-analysis**).

Positive predictive value – proportion of people with a positive test who have the target disorder (*see also* **Likelihood ratio**).

Randomised controlled clinical trial (RCT) – a group of patients is randomised into an experimental group and a control group. These groups are followed up for the variables / outcomes of interest (*see also* **Review of study designs**).

Relative risk reduction (RRR) – *see* **Treatment effects**.

Risk ratio (RR) – is the ratio of risk in the treated group (EER) to the risk in the control group (CER) – used in randomised trials and cohort studies:

$$RR = ERR/CER$$

Sensitivity – proportion of people with the target disorder who have a positive test. It is used to assist in assessing and selecting a diagnostic test/sign/symptom (*see also* **Likelihood ratio**).

SnNout – when a sign/test/symptom has a high **S**ensitivity, a **N**egative result rules **out** the diagnosis, e.g. the sensitivity of a history of ankle swelling for diagnosing ascites is 93%, therefore if a person does not have a history of ankle swelling, it is highly unlikely that the person has ascites.

Specificity – proportion of people without the target disorder who have a negative test. It is used to assist in assessing and selecting a diagnostic test/sign/symptom (*see also* **Likelihood ratio**).

SpPin – when a sign/test/symptom has a high **S**pecificity, a **P**ositive result rules **in** the diagnosis, e.g. the specificity of a fluid wave for diagnosing ascites is 92%, therefore if a person does have a fluid wave, it rules in the diagnosis of ascites

Systematic review – *see* **Overview**.

Treatment effects
The E-B journals have achieved consensus on some terms they use to describe both the good and the bad effects of therapy. They will join the terms already in current use (RRR, ARR, NNT), and both sets are described here and summarised in the Glossary that appears inside the back cover of *Evidence-based Medicine*. We will bring them to life with a synthesis of three randomised trials in diabetes which individually showed that several years of intensive insulin therapy reduced the proportion of patients with worsening retinopathy to 13% from 38%, raised the proportion of patients with satisfactory haemoglobin A1c levels to 60% from about 30%, and increased the proportion of patients with at least one episode of symptomatic hypoglycaemia to 47% from 23%. Note that in each case the first number constitutes the 'experimental event rate' or EER and the second number the 'control

event rate' or CER. We will use the following terms and calculations to describe these effects of treatment:

When the experimental treatment reduces the probability of a bad outcome (worsening diabetic retinopathy).

RRR (Relative risk reduction): the proportional reduction in rates of bad outcomes between experimental and control participants in a trial, calculated as IEER − CERI/CER, and accompanied by a 95% confidence interval (CI). In the case of worsening diabetic retinopathy, IEE − CERI/CER = I13% − 38%I/38% = 66%.

ARR (Absolute risk reduction): the absolute arithmetic difference in rates of bad outcomes between experimental and control participants in a trial, calculated as IEER − CERI, and accompanied by a 95% CI. In this case, IEER − CERI = I13% − 38%I = 25%.

NNT (Number needed to treat): the number of patients who need to be treated to achieve 1 additional favourable outcome, calculated as 1/ARR and accompanied by a 95% CI. In this case, 1/ARR = 1/25% = 4.

Calculations for the occurrence of diabetic retinopathy in IDDMs:

Occurrence of diabetic neuropathy at 5 yr among insulin-dependent diabetics in the DCCT trial		Relative risk reduction (RRR)	Absolute risk reduction (ARR)	Number needed to treat (NNT)
Usual insulin regimen CER	Intensive insulin regimen EER	$\dfrac{\text{IEER} - \text{CERI}}{\text{CER}}$	IEER − CERI	1/ARR
13%	38%	$\dfrac{\text{I}13\% - 38\%\text{I}}{38\%} = 66\%$	I13% − 38%I = 25%	1/25% = 4 pts, for 6 years, with intensive insulin Rx

When the experimental treatment increases the probability of a good outcome (satisfactory haemoglobin A1c levels).

RBI (Relative benefit increase): the proportional increase in rates of good outcomes between experimental and control patients in a trial, calculated as IEER-CERI/CER, and accompanied by a 95% confidence interval (CI). In the case of satisfactory haemoglobin A1c levels, IEER − CERI/CER = I60% − 30%I/30% = 100%.

ABI (Absolute benefit increase): the absolute arithmetic difference in rates of good outcomes between experimental and control patients in a trial, calculated as IEER − CERI, and accompanied by a 95% CI. In the case of satisfactory haemoglobin A1c levels, IEER − CERI = I60% − 30%I = 30%.

NNT (Number needed to treat): The number of patients who need to be treated to achieve one additional good outcome, calculated as 1/ARR and accompanied by a 95% CI. In this case, 1/ARR = 1/30% = 3.

When the experimental treatment increase the probability of a bad outcome (episodes of hypoglycaemia).

RRI (Relative risk increase): the proportional increase in rates of bad outcomes between experimental and control patients in a trial, calculated as |EER – CER|/CER, and accompanied by a 95% CI. In the case of hypoglycaemic episodes, |EER – CER|/CER = |57% – 23%|/57% = 34%/57% = 60%. (RRI is also used in assessing the impact of 'risk factors' for disease.)

ARI (Absolute risk increase): the absolute arithmetic difference in rates of bad outcomes between experimental and control patients in a trial, calculated as |EER – CER|, and accompanied by a 95% CI. In the case of hypoglycaemic episodes, |EER – CER| = |57% – 23%| = 34%. (ARI is also used in assessing the impact of 'risk factors' for disease.)

NNH (Number needed to harm): the number of patients who, if they received the experimental treatment, would lead to one additional patient being harmed, compared with patients who received the control treatment, calculated as 1/ARR and accompanied by a 95% CI. In this case, 1/ARR = 1/34% = 3.

	Adverse Outcome		Totals
	Present (case)	**Absent (control)**	
Exposed to the Treatment — Yes (cohort)	a	b	a+b
No (cohort)	c	d	c+d
Totals	a+c	b+d	a+b+c+d

In a randomised trial or cohort study:
Relative risk = RR = [a/(a+b)]/[c/(c+d)]

In a case-control study:
Odds ratio (or Relative odds) = OR = ad/bc

Randomized controlled trial: start with a+b+c+d and randomise to (a+b) and (c+d)

Advantages

1   Assignment to treatment can be kept concealed.

2   Confounders equally distributed.

3   Blinding more likely.

4   Randomisation facilitates statistical analysis.

Disadvantages

1   Expensive – time and money.

2   Volunteer bias.

3   Ethically problematic at times.

Crossover design

Advantages

1   Subjects serve as own controls and error variance is reduced thus reducing sample size needed.

2   All subjects receive treatment (at least some of the time).

3   Statistical tests assuming randomisation can be used.

4   Blinding can be maintained.

Disadvantages

1   All subjects receive placebo or alternative treatment at some point.

2   Washout period lengthy or unknown.

3   Cannot be used for treatments with permanent effects.

Cohort study: selects (a+b) and (c+d)

Advantages

1 Ethically safe.

2 Subjects can be matched.

3 Can establish timing and directionality of events.

4 Eligibility criteria and outcome assessments can be standardised.

5 Administratively easier and cheaper than RCT.

Disadvantages

1 Controls may be difficult to identify.

2 Exposure may be linked to a hidden confounder.

3 Blinding difficult.

4 Still expensive.

5 Randomisation not present.

6 For rare disease, large sample sizes or long follow-up necessary.

Cross-sectional (analytic) survey: selecting a+b+c+d

Advantages

1 Cheap and simple.

2 Safe ethically.

Disadvantages

1 Establishes association at most, not causality.

2 Recall bias susceptibility.

3 Confounders may be unequally distributed.

4 Neyman bias.

5 Group sizes may be unequal.

Case-control study: selecting (a+c) and (b+d)

Advantages

1 Quick and cheap.

2 Only feasible method for very rare disorders or those with long lag between exposure and outcome.

3 Fewer subjects needed than cross-sectional studies.

Disadvantages

1 Reliance on recall or records to determine exposure status.

2 Confounders.

3 Selection of control groups difficult.

4 Potential bias – recall, selection.

Section 3a1

Is this evidence about a diagnostic test valid?

Having found a possibly useful article about a diagnostic test, how can you quickly critically appraise it for its proximity to the truth? This can be done by asking some simple questions; often you'll find their answers in the article's abstract. Table 3a1.1 lists these questions for individual reports, but you can also apply them to the interpretation of a systematic review (overview) of several different studies of the same diagnostic test for the same target disorder.*

The first guide is: 'Was there an independent, blind comparison with a reference ("gold") standard of diagnosis?' This is quite a mouthful, but it simply means that two criteria should have been met. The patients in the study should have undergone *both* the diagnostic test in question (say, an item of the history or physical examination, a blood test, etc.) *and* the reference (or 'gold') standard (an autopsy or biopsy or other confirmatory 'proof' that they do or don't have the target disorder); and the results of one shouldn't be known to those who are applying and interpreting the other (for example, the pathologist interpreting the biopsy that comprises the reference standard for the target disorder should be 'blind' to the result of the blood test that comprises the diagnostic test under study). In this way, investigators avoid the conscious and unconscious bias that otherwise might cause the reference standard to be 'overinterpreted' when the diagnostic test is positive and 'underinterpreted' when it is negative. Sometimes investigators have a difficult time coming up with clearcut

* As we'll stress throughout this book, systematic reviews will give you the most valid and useful external evidence on just about any clinical question you can pose. They are still pretty rare for diagnostic tests and for this reason we'll describe them in their usual, therapeutic habitat, in Section 3a3. When using Table 3a3.2 to consider diagnostic tests, simply substitute 'diagnostic test' for 'treatment' as you read.

Table 3a1.1 Are the results of this diagnostic study valid?

1. Was there an independent, blind comparison with a reference ('gold') standard of diagnosis?
2. Was the diagnostic test evaluated in an appropriate spectrum of patients (like those in whom it would be used in practice)?
3. Was the reference standard applied regardless of the diagnostic test result?

reference standards (e.g. for psychiatric disorders) and you'll want to give careful consideration to their arguments justifying the selection of their reference standard.

One way or another, the report will wind up calling some results 'normal' and others 'abnormal' and we'll show you how to interpret these in Section 3b1. For now, you might simply want to recognize that there are six definitions of 'normal' in common use (we've listed them in Table 3a1.2). We will make use of definition 5 ('diagnostic' normal) and believe that half of the definitions are not useful. The first two (the Gaussian and percentile definitions) are derived from the study test results alone, with no reference standard, and simply define the 'normal range' for the diagnostic test result on the basis of statistical properties (standard deviations or percentiles). Thus they are properties of the test in isolation from any objective reality. These don't make any sense to us, for they imply that all 'abnormalities' occur at the same frequency. They both suggest that if we can perform enough diagnostic tests on a patient we are bound to find something 'abnormal' and lead to all sorts of inappropriate further testing. The third definition of 'normal' (culturally desirable) represents a cultural value judgment. It is seen in fashion advertisements and at the fringes of the 'lifestyle' movement where medicine becomes confused with morality. The fourth (risk factor) definition has the drawback that it 'labels' or stigmatizes some patients and is clinically useful only if we can do something positive to lower their risk. The fifth (diagnostic) definition is the one that we will focus on here and we will show you how to generate and interpret diagnostic normality in Section 3b1. The final (therapeutic) definition is in part an outgrowth of the

Table 3a1.2 Six definitions of normal

1. Gaussian: the mean +/- 2 standard deviations. Assumes a normal distribution and means that all 'abnormalities' have the same frequency.
2. Percentile: within the range, say, of 5–95%. Has the same basic defect as the Gaussian definition.
3. Culturally desirable: preferred by society. Confuses the role of medicine.
4. Risk factor: carrying no additional risk of disease. Labels the outliers, who may not be helped.
5. Diagnostic: range of results beyond which target disorders become highly probable – the focus of this discussion.
6. Therapeutic: range of results beyond which treatment does more good than harm. Means you have to keep up with advances in therapy!

fourth (risk factor) definition and has the great clinical advantage that it changes with our knowledge of efficacy. Thus, the definition of normal blood pressure has changed radically over the past few decades as we have learned that treatment of progressively lower blood pressure levels does more good than harm.

Returning to the second question in Table 3a1.1, you will want the diagnostic test to have been evaluated in an appropriate spectrum of patients, similar to the practice population in which the test might be used. Among patients with late or severe disease, when the diagnosis is obvious, often you won't need any diagnostic test, so studies that confine themselves to florid cases are not very informative. The article will be informative if the diagnostic test was applied to patients with mild as well as severe and early as well as late cases of the target disorder and among both treated and untreated individuals. In addition, you would want the diagnostic test to have been applied to patients with different disorders that are commonly confused with the target disorder of interest.

Finally, was the reference standard applied regardless of the diagnostic test result? When patients have a negative diagnostic test result, investigators are tempted to forego applying the reference standard and when the latter is invasive or risky (e.g. angiography) it may be considered inappropriate

Section 3a2

Is this evidence about prognosis valid?

Clinicians consider questions about prognosis all the time. Sometimes the questions are posed by patients and are quite direct (How long have I got?). At other times the questions are posed by clinicians and are indirect, as when deciding *whether* to treat at all (e.g. an elderly man with chronic lymphocyte leukemia who feels well – would his prognosis be importantly altered if he were left alone until he becomes symptomatic?) or deciding *whether* to screen (e.g. for abdominal aortic aneurysms – what is the fate of the undetected 4 cm aneurysm?). These questions share two elements: a qualitative aspect (Which outcomes could happen?) and a temporal aspect (Over what time period?). In Chapter 1 we showed you how to recognize such questions as being about prognosis and in Chapter 2 we addressed how to find good information about prognosis. In this part of Chapter 3 we'll present a framework for appraising the validity and importance of evidence about prognosis, for use when you tackle situations like the ones above (see Table 3a2.1). We'll consider them in sequence.

The four guides that will help you decide whether some evidence about prognosis is valid are listed in Table 3a2.1. First of all, was a defined, representative sample of patients assembled at a common (usually early) point in the course of their disease? Ideally, the prognosis study you find would include the entire population of patients who ever lived who developed the disease, studied from the instant of its onset. Since this is impossible, you'll want to look at how far from ideal will still tell you what you need to know and you'll do that by finding the methods section (if there isn't one, maybe you're wasting your time on this report!) and reading how the study patients were assembled. You'd want their illness to be defined well enough for you to be clear about it and you'd want the entire spectrum of severity that would occur at that common point to be represented.

But when should the 'clock start'? That is, from what point in the disease should patients be followed? If investigators begin tracking outcomes only *after* several patients have already finished their course with the disease, then the outcomes for these patients would never be counted. Some would have recovered quickly, whilst others might have died quickly. So, to avoid missing outcomes by 'starting the clock' too late, you should look to see that study patients were included at a uniformly early time in the disease, ideally when it first becomes clinically manifest, the so-called 'inception cohort'. An exception might be if you wanted to learn about the prognosis of a late stage in the disease (e.g. for clinically manifest coronary heart disease); in this case you'd look for a representative and well-defined sample of patients who were all at a similarly advanced stage (e.g. when they had their first clinical coronary event, not when they first developed elevated coronary risk factors).

Second, was patient follow-up sufficiently long and complete? Ideally, every patient in the inception cohort would be followed over time until they fully recover or one of the disease outcomes occurs. If with short follow-up few study patients have any of the outcomes of interest, you won't have enough to go on when advising your patients. Of course, if after decades of follow-up few adverse events have occurred, this good prognostic result is very useful in reassuring your patient about the future. If you think that the follow-up is too short to have developed a valid picture of the extent of the outcome of your interest, you'd better look for other evidence.

---

to do so. For this reason, many investigators now employ a reference standard for a patient *not* having the target disorder in which they *don't* suffer any adverse health outcome during a long follow-up on no definitive treatment (for example, convincing evidence that a patient with clinically suspected deep vein thrombosis did *not* have this disorder would be a prolonged follow-up on no antithrombotic therapy and suffering no ill effects).

If the report you're reading fails one or more of these three tests you'll need to consider whether it has a fatal flaw that renders its conclusions invalid; if so, it's back to more searching (either now or later; if you haven't enough time, perhaps you can interest a colleague or trainee in taking this on). If the report passes this initial scrutiny and you decide that you can believe its results, but you haven't already carried out the second critical appraisal step of deciding whether these results are impressive, then you can proceed to Section 3b1 on page 118.

Further reading

Jaeschke R, Guyatt G H, Sackett D L for the Evidence-Based Medicine Working Group. Users' guides to the medical literature. VI. How to use an article about a diagnostic test. A: Are the results of the study valid? JAMA 1994; 271: 389–91.

Table 3a2.1 Is this evidence about prognosis valid?

1. Was a defined, representative sample of patients assembled at a common (usually early) point in the course of their disease?
2. Was patient follow-up sufficiently long and complete?
3. Were objective outcome criteria applied in a 'blind' fashion?
4. If subgroups with different prognoses are identified:
   ● Was there adjustment for important prognostic factors?
   ● Was there validation in an independent group of 'test-set' patients?

If follow-up was long enough, you still have to worry about patients who entered the study but got lost along the way. Patients are almost always lost to follow-up and their outcomes will be excluded from the study's conclusions about prognosis. Some losses to follow-up are both unavoidable and unrelated to prognosis (e.g. moving away to a better job) and these aren't a cause for worry. But other losses might be because patients die or are too ill to continue follow-up (or lose their independence and move in with family) and the failure to document and report their outcomes will threaten the validity of the report. Short of finding a report that kept track of every patient, how can you judge whether follow-up is 'sufficiently complete'? There is no single answer for all studies, but we offer two suggestions to help you make this judgment. The first is a simple '5 and 20' rule of thumb: fewer than 5% loss probably leads to little bias, greater than 20% loss seriously threatens validity and in-between amounts cause intermediate amounts of trouble. While this may be easy to remember, it may oversimplify for clinical situations in which the outcomes are infrequent.

The second approach uses a 'worst-case' scenario. Imagine a study of prognosis wherein 100 patients enter the study, four die and 16 are lost to follow-up. A 'crude' survival rate would count the four deaths among the 84 with total follow-up, for a death rate of 4.8%, and then report a survival rate of $100\% - 4.8\% = 95.2\%$. But what of the lost 16? Some or all of them might have died too. The latter, 'worst-case' scenario would mean a case-fatality rate of (four known + 16 lost) or 20 out of (84 followed up + 16 lost) or 20/100, that is 20% (four times the observed rate); note that in order to determine the 'worst-case' scenario you've added the lost patients to both the numerator and denominator of the outcome rate. On the other hand, in the 'best-case' scenario none of the lost 16 would have died, yielding a case-fatality rate of 4 out of (84 + 16) or 4/100, that is 4%; note that in determining the 'best-case' scenario you add the missing cases to just the denominator. While this 'best case' of 4% may not differ much from the observed 4.8%, the 'worst case' of 20% does differ meaningfully and you'd probably judge that this study's follow-up

was not sufficiently complete. By seeing what effect the losses might have on the result you can decide whether a 'worst-case' scenario would change your conclusion about prognosis. If this simple form of 'sensitivity analysis' suggests that losses wouldn't change the result much, then you can judge the follow-up as sufficiently complete.

You can use these first two guides to screen articles about prognosis to find the few worth more of your limited time. If you've answered 'no' to both of the above questions, you can be pretty sure the study will not provide estimates of prognosis that are close to the truth and you ought to start searching for better evidence. If, on the other hand, you've answered 'yes' to both of the above questions, you can be reasonably confident that the study will provide accurate information about prognosis. To be even more sure of this, you should ask the remaining two validity questions in Table 3a2.1.

Were objective outcome criteria applied in a 'blind' fashion? Diseases can affect patients in many important ways; some are easy to spot and some are more subtle. In general, outcomes at both extremes, death or full recovery, are relatively easy to detect and be sure of. In between these extremes are a wide range of outcomes that can be more difficult to detect or confirm and where investigators will have to use judgment in deciding how to count them up. Examples include the degree of disease activity/quiescence, the readiness for return to work and the intensity of residual pain. To minimize the effects of bias, investigators can establish specific criteria that define each possible outcome of the disease and then use these criteria during patient follow-up. You can usually find such outcome criteria in the text, tables, appendices or references in the study. You should satisfy yourself that they are sufficiently objective for confirming the outcomes you're interested in. The occurrence of death is about as objective as you can get, but judging the underlying cause of death is very prone to error (especially when it's based on death certificates) and can be biased unless objective criteria are applied to high-quality clinical evidence.

But even with objective criteria, some bias might creep in if the investigators judging the outcomes also know the

patients' characteristics. To minimize this bias, the authors of the report should have taken precautions so that the investigators making judgments about clinical outcomes were 'blind' to these patients' clinical characteristics and prognostic factors. The more subjective the outcome, the more important such blinding becomes. You should satisfy yourself that blinding was used if it would have been important for the outcomes of interest to you.

The final pair of guides have to do with reports that claim that one subgroup of patients has a different prognosis from others. Such reports are common and for good clinical reason. Often you will want to know whether subgroups of patients have different prognoses (e.g. among patients with non-valvular atrial fibrillation, are those with enlarged left atria at higher risk for stroke than those with normal sized atria?). The first guide here suggests that you look to see whether there was adjustment for other important prognostic factors. That is, reports that address this sort of question should have made sure that these subgroup predictions aren't being distorted by the unequal occurrence of another, powerful prognostic factor (such as would occur if patients with large atria were also more likely to have had prior embolic stroke than patients with normal atria). There are both simple (e.g. stratified analyses displaying the prognoses of patients with large atria separately for those with and without prior embolic stroke) and fancy (e.g. multiple regression analyses that could take into account not only prior embolic stroke but also hypertension, left ventricular function and the like) ways of adjusting for these other important prognostic factors and you should reassure yourself that one or the other has been applied before you tentatively accept the conclusion about a different prognosis for the subgroup of interest.

We say tentatively because there is one final guide to deciding whether a claim that a subgroup has a different prognosis should be accepted as valid. This is the fact that the statistics of determining subgroup prognoses are all about prediction, not explanation. They are indifferent to whether the prognostic factor is physiologically logical (in our running example, left atrial size) or biologically nonsensical (whether the

Evidence-based Medicine

patient's navel is concave (an 'innie') or convex (an 'outie'). These prognostic factors can be demographic (such as age, gender, socioeconomic status), disease specific (such as extent of disease, degree of test abnormality) or comorbid (presence or absence of many other conditions). Keep in mind that these prognostic factors need not cause the outcome; they need only be associated with its development strongly enough to predict it.

For this reason, the first time a prognostic factor is identified, there is no guarantee it isn't the result of a random, non-causal 'quirk' in its distribution between patients with different prognoses; for that reason, the initial patient group in which it was identified is called a 'training set'. As you might imagine, if this initial study carried out a multivariate analysis looking for potential prognostic factors, they'd be very likely to find at least a few, just on the basis of chance (and most investigators would be imaginative enough to suggest logical explanations for them). Because of this risk of spurious, chance nomination of prognostic factors, you should seek its confirmation in a report of a second, independent group (called a 'test set') of patients. The best evidence for this is finding a statement (in the methods section) of a prestudy intention to examine this specific possible prognostic factor (based on its appearance in a training set). If that second, independent study also identifies the prognostic factor, you can feel much more confident that the evidence about it is valid.

If your evidence flunks these tests for validity, we're afraid it's back to searching, either now (if you still have time) or at a later session. If, on a happier note, you decide that the evidence you've found about a prognostic factor is valid and you haven't already decided whether it's also important, you can take that consideration up in Section 3b2 on page 129.

Further reading

Laupacis A, Wells G, Richardson W S, Tugwell P for the Evidence-Based Medicine Working Group. Users' guides to the medical literature. V. How to use an article about prognosis. JAMA 1994; 272: 234–7.

Table 3a3.1 Are the results of this single study valid?

The main questions to answer:
1. Was the assignment of patients to treatments randomized? and was the randomization list concealed?
2. Were all patients who entered the trial accounted for at its conclusion? and were they analyzed in the groups to which they were randomized?

And some finer points to address:
1. Were patients and clinicians kept 'blind' to which treatment was being received?
2. Aside from the experimental treatment, were the groups treated equally?
3. Were the groups similar at the start of the trial?

Section 3a3

Is this evidence about a treatment valid?

Having found some possibly useful evidence about therapy, you have to decide where to start in its critical appraisal. On the one hand, you could start here in Section 3a3, with an appraisal of its validity (arguing that if it's not valid, who cares whether it appears to show a big effect?). On the other, you could go right to determining its importance in Section 3b3 (arguing that if the evidence doesn't suggest a possibly useful clinical impact, who cares if it's valid?). Begin with either and then pick up the other. This section will help you to quickly and critically appraise evidence about therapy for its closeness to the truth. This can be done by asking some simple questions and often you'll find their answers in an abstract that accompanies the evidence. Table 3a3.1 lists these questions for reports of individual therapeutic trials, but since these can best be interpreted in the context of all other trials on the same topic, Table 3a3.2 summarizes guides for assessing evidence that has combined the results of several trials into an overview or systematic review (when a systematic review uses special statistical methods for combining the results of several studies, we call it a meta-analysis). Alternatively, you may encounter (or have tracked down) an economic analysis, which is a more complex method that compares therapeutic alternatives from a broader perspective (including those of health managers or even society as a whole) and tries to offer or provide treatments in the way that best uses scarce resources such as hospital beds, drugs, operating time, clinicians and money. Questions pertinent to deciding whether you should believe an economic analysis appear in Table 3a3.3. Finally, and building on the earlier section on diagnosis, we'll give you a brief description of how to decide whether to believe evidence on the effects of therapy when it is formulated into a clinical decision analysis; rules for deciding whether to believe their results are described in Section 3a3.4.

When several randomized trials of the same treatment for the same condition have been carried out, we think you'll agree that an overview which systematically reviews and combines all of them would give you a better answer than a critical appraisal of just one of them. For that reason, we suggested back in Chapter 2 that you always start your search for useful clinical articles on just about any topic by looking for systematic reviews. However, because systematic reviews assess their component trials individually (and, as you can see in Table 3a3.2, you want to be sure that they've done that in a valid way) and since at this point in history you're much more likely to find individual trials than systematic reviews, we'll begin with the individual trial.

Is the evidence from this randomized trial valid?

We'll begin with two important questions:

1. Was the assignment of patients to treatments randomized and was the randomization schedule concealed?

When deciding whether the evidence from a randomized trial is valid, the most important question to ask (and frequently the quickest question to answer) is: Was the assignment of patients to treatments randomized? That is, was some method analogous to tossing a coin* used to assign patients to treatments (with the treatment you're interested in given if the coin landed 'heads' and a conventional, 'control' or placebo† treatment given if the coin landed 'tails')? The reason for insisting on random allocation to treatments is that this comes closer than any other research design to creating groups of patients at the start of the trial who are identical in their risk of the events you're hoping to prevent. It does this in two, related ways. First, the coin toss balances the groups for prognostic factors (such as disease severity or other predictors of especially good or bad prognosis) which, if they were unevenly distributed between treatment groups, could exaggerate, cancel or even counteract the effects of therapy.‡ If they exaggerated the apparent effects of an otherwise ineffectual treatment, the effects of their imbalance could lead to the false-positive conclusion that the treatment was useful when it was not. And if they cancelled or counteracted the effects of a really efficacious treatment, the effects of their imbalance could lead to the false-negative conclusions that a useful treatment was useless or even harmful. Random allocation balances the treatment groups for these and other prognostic factors, even if we don't yet understand the disorder well enough to know what they are!

The second, related benefit of random allocation is that, if it is concealed from the clinicians who are entering patients into the trial, they will be unaware of which treatment the next patient will receive and they can't either consciously or unconsciously distort the balance between the groups being compared. So you want to be sure that both of these standards are met. Usually it's easy to tell whether a study was

* In practice, this coin tossing is done by special computer programs, but the principle is exactly the same.
† A placebo is a treatment that is so similar in appearance, taste, etc. that the patient ('single-blind') or the clinician or both ('double-blind') are unable to distinguish it from the active treatment.
‡ 'Confounder' is a technical name for these sorts of patient characteristics that are extraneous to the question posed, could cause the clinical events we are trying to prevent with the treatment and might be unevenly distributed between the treatment groups. And although there are other ways of avoiding confounding (exclusion, stratified sampling, matching, stratified analysis, standardization and multivariate modelling), they all demand that you already know what the confounder is.

randomized, because it's something to be proud of and that term often appears in the title and almost always in the abstract. On the other hand, it's not often stated whether the randomization list was concealed, but if randomization occurred by telephone or by some system that was at a distance from where patients were being entered into the trial, you can be comfortable about this. If randomization wasn't concealed, this tends to lead to patients with more favourable prognoses being given the experimental treatment, exaggerating the apparent benefits of therapy and perhaps even leading to the false-positive conclusion that the treatment is efficacious when it is not.

If you find that the study was not randomized, we'd suggest that you stop reading it and go on to the next article. Only if you can't find any randomized trials should you come back and have another go at it. But if the only evidence you have about a treatment is from non-randomized studies, you are in a bind and have five options:

1. Check Chapter 2 again or get help in doing another literature search to see if you missed any randomized trials of the candidate therapy.

2. See whether the treatment effect is simply so huge that you can't imagine it could be a false-positive study (this usually happens only when the prognosis is uniformly awful and is a very rare situation). As a check, ask several colleagues whether they consider the candidate therapy so likely to be efficacious that they'd consider it unethical to randomize a patient like yours into a study of it that includes a no-treatment or placebo group.*

3. Conversely, if the non-randomized study concluded that the treatment was useless or harmful, then it is usually safe to accept that conclusion (since, as described above, false-negative conclusions from non-randomized studies are less likely than false-positive ones).

4. Consider whether an 'N-of-1' trial would make sense to you and your patient (they are described on page 173).

* This is the 'convincing non-experimental evidence' category used in the audits of clinical care reported on page 3 (the A-team study).

5. Try some other treatment or simply provide supportive care.

2. Were all patients who entered the trial accounted for at its conclusion and were they analysed in the groups to which they were randomized?

Having satisfied yourself that the trial really was randomized, you can then match the number of patients who entered the trial with the number accounted for at its conclusion. Ideally, these numbers will be identical, for lost patients could have had events that would change the conclusion. If, for example, patients on the experimental treatment dropped out and had adverse outcomes, their absence from the analysis would lead it to overestimate the efficacy of that treatment. What's an acceptable loss? To be sure of a trial's conclusion, its authors should be able to take all patients who were lost along the way, assign them the 'worst-case' outcomes (that is, assume that everyone lost from the group whose remaining members fared better had a bad outcome and assume that everyone lost from the group whose remaining members fared worse had a rosy outcome) and still be able to support their original conclusion. It would be unusual for a trial to withstand a worst-case analysis if it lost more than 20% of its patients and journals like *Evidence-Based Medicine* won't publish trials with <80% follow-up.

Because anything that happens after randomization can affect the chances that a patient in a trial has an event, it's important that all patients (even those who fail to take their medicine or accidentally or intentionally receive the wrong treatment) are analysed in the groups to which they were randomized. This is an essential prerequisite for valid evidence about the effects of therapy. For example, it has repeatedly been shown that patients who do and don't take their study medicine have very different outcomes, even when the study medicine they have been prescribed is a placebo! The correct form of analysis, in which patients are analysed in the groups to which they were assigned, is called an 'intention to treat' analysis.

There are three less important questions to ask when you are trying to decide whether a randomized trial has produced valid evidence:

1. Were patients and clinicians kept 'blind' to which treatment was being received?

2. Aside from the experimental treatment, were the groups treated equally?

3. Were the groups similar at the start of the trial?

If you decide that the study really was randomized, follow-up was virtually complete and patients were analyzed in the groups to which they'd been randomized, you can look for some other features that provide even greater assurance that you can believe its results. If, for example, it was a pharmacological trial in which patients received either a tablet containing the active drug or an identical-appearing (in size, shape, colour, taste, etc.) tablet of pharmacologically inert ingredients (a placebo), then it would be possible to keep both patients and clinicians blind* as to which treatment was received and neither the patient's reporting of symptoms nor the clinician's interpretation of them would be influenced by their hunches about whether the treatment was efficacious. Another advantage of the double-blind method is that it prevents patients and their clinicians from adding any additional treatments (or 'cointerventions') to just one of the groups. When patients and their clinicians can't be kept blind (as in surgical trials), often it is possible to have other, blinded clinicians come in and assess clinical records (purged of any mention of treatment) or make special outcome measurements. And finally, you can double-check to see whether randomization was effective by looking to see whether patients were similar at the start of the trial (most trials display this in the first table of their results).

Whether the results of an individual trial are important is considered in Section 3b3 on page 133.

* When patients don't know their treatment but their doctors do (as when the active drug causes a clearcut sign such as bradycardia), the trial is called 'single blind'. When both are blind, it is called 'double blind'.

Is the evidence from this systematic review valid?

Having shown you how to decide whether to believe the results of a single trial, let's now turn to how you can decide whether to believe the results of an overview of several trials. The key questions you need to answer are in Table 3a3.2.

Table 3a3.2 Are the results of this systematic review valid?

1. Is it an overview of randomized trials of the treatment you're interested in?
2. Does it include a methods section that describes:
   a. finding and including all the relevant trials?
   b. assessing their individual validity?
3. Were the results consistent from study to study?

1. Is it a systematic review of randomized trials of the treatment you're interested in?

This first question asks whether you are sure that the treatment is the same as the one you're considering and immediately asking whether the overview is combining reports of studies carried out at the same, most powerful level of evidence that we've been discussing here, the randomized trial. Systematic reviews of non-randomized studies of therapy simply compound the problems of individually misleading trials and the same warnings apply. Moreover, some overviews combine randomized and non-randomized studies and unless the authors have provided separate information on the subset of randomized trials, you shouldn't trust them either.

2. Does it include a methods section that describes: (a) finding and including all the relevant trials; (b) assessing their individual validity?

You should see whether the overview report includes a methods section that describes how they found all the relevant trials and how they assessed their individual validity. Let's take these three elements one by one. First, because performing an overview is performing research (it involves posing a question, identifying a population and drawing a sample, making measurements, analyzing them and drawing

conclusions), it should be carried out and reported like research. If you don't find a methods section, be very wary of believing its results; maybe its only useful part will be its bibliography of individual trials for you to study as above. Second, if the overview has a methods section it should describe how its authors tracked down and included all the trials that were relevant to this treatment. This is no easy task. The standard bibliographic databases described in Chapter 2. good as they are, fail to correctly label up to half of the published trials and 'negative' trials (that conclude the treatment is not efficacious) are less likely to be submitted for publication, leading an overview of those that are published to overestimate the treatment's efficacy. Signs that the overviewers did a good job are positive when they report at least some hand searching of the most relevant journals (for miscoded trials) and especially when they report contacting the authors of published trials (who often will know about unpublished ones). Third, you should look for a statement of how they decided whether the individual trials in their overview were scientifically sound, using criteria like those in Table 3a3.1. Finally, because these last two steps of deciding which trials to include in the overview involve a lot of judgment calls, you should be especially reassured when you find that two or more investigators carried out these tasks independent of each other and achieved good agreement about their judgments.

3. Were the results consistent from study to study?

It stands to reason that we are more likely to believe an overview when the results of all the trials in it show a treatment effect going in the same direction. Although we shouldn't expect each of them to show exactly the same degree of efficacy (that is, we should be comfortable with a certain amount of quantitative difference in the trial results), we would be concerned if we found some trials in an overview confidently concluding a beneficial effect of the treatment and other trials confidently concluding no benefit or a harmful effect. Such a qualitative difference in the effects of treatment (which also goes by the name of heterogeneity), unless it can be explained to your satisfaction (such as by differences in patients or in doses or durations of treatment), should lead you to be very cautious about believing any overall conclusion about efficacy in all patients and you'd hope to see your caution expressed in the conclusions of the overview.

Whether the results of an overview are important is considered in Section 3b3 on page 133.

Section 3a4

Is this evidence about harm valid?

You must frequently make judgments on whether a treatment is harming or has harmed a patient. Many admissions to acute general hospitals are the result of adverse drug reactions and reactions to diagnostic and therapeutic maneuvers are judged to befall one-fifth to one-third of patients after they are admitted. On the other hand, even clinical pharmacologists disagree about whether a given patient has had an adverse drug reaction and the fact that an adverse reaction occurred *during* a treatment is insufficient evidence that it occurred *because* of that treatment.

Faced with a problem that is pandemic yet controvertible, clinicians must equip themselves to answer two related questions:

1. Does this drug (or operation or other treatment) cause that adverse effect in *some* patients? And, if so:
2. Did this drug (or operation or other treatment) cause that adverse effect in *this particular* patient?

This section will deal with the first question and the second question will be addressed in Section 4.4.

Because this assessment can be viewed as addressing a general question of *causation*, it benefits from what has been learned about asking and answering such questions in classical epidemiology. The four guides for deciding whether to believe the claim that a treatment harms some patients are summarized in Table 3a4.1, and we'll consider them in sequence.

1. Were there clearly defined groups of patients, similar in all important ways other than exposure to the treatment?

Because the 'threats to validity' are different for different sorts of studies, you'll have to spend just a little time sorting them out. Suppose you wanted to decide whether fenoterol (a beta-agonist used to treat asthma) sometimes (albeit

Table 3a4.1 Are the results of this harm study valid?

1. Were there clearly defined groups of patients, similar in all important ways other than exposure to the treatment?
2. Were treatment exposures and clinical outcomes measured in the same way in both groups?
3. Was the follow-up of study patients complete and long enough?
4. Do the results satisfy some 'diagnostic tests for causation'?
   - Is it clear that the exposure preceded the onset of the outcome?
   - Is there a dose-response gradient?
   - Is there positive evidence from a 'dechallenge-rechallenge' study?
   - Is the association consistent from study to study?
   - Does the association make biological sense?

rarely) caused the death of its users. You could look for and find four different sorts of studies and all of them can be illustrated by reference to Table 3a4.2. First, you could look for a randomized trial in which asthma patients were assigned, by a system analogous to tossing a coin, to receive fenoterol (the top row in Table 3a4.2, whose total is **a+b**)

	Adverse Outcome		Totals
	Present (Case)	Absent (Control)	
Exposed to the treatment — Yes (Cohort)	a	b	a+b
Exposed to the treatment — No (Cohort)	c	d	c+d
Totals	a+c	b+d	a+b+c+d

Table 3a4.2 Different ways of finding out whether a treatment sometimes causes harm

or some comparison treatment or placebo (the bottom row, whose total is **c+d**). Since the randomization would make them similar for all other features that would cause their deaths, you'd be pretty likely to judge any statistically significant increase in deaths among fenoterol recipients (cell **a**) as valid. Trouble is, if fenoterol causes only one extra death per 1000 users, you'd have to find an awfully big trial to show a clear excess among fenoterol-treated asthmatics. As it happens, if a drug causes an adverse reaction once per x patients who receive it (say, once per 1000), to be 95% certain to see at least one adverse reaction you need to follow 3x patients (in this example, 3000). For that reason, you usually can't find the most valid data on harm from individual randomized trials and if you can't find a systematic review with a large enough total number of patients to suffice, you'll have to work with non-experimental evidence.

The next most powerful design is also conducted along the rows of Table 3a4.2, but this time the groups of patients (called 'cohorts') who are (**a+b**) and are not (**c+d**) exposed to the treatment are formed not by random allocation, but by the decisions of clinicians and patients to have some of them ('exposed') receive the treatment and others ('unexposed') not receive it. These cohorts are then followed to determine which and how many of them develop the bad outcome (**a or c**). As you can see, there is no reason why these cohorts should be otherwise perfectly identical to each other and plenty of reason for them to be quite different (e.g. sicker patients who are more likely to have adverse outcomes might be more likely to be offered a 'last-ditch' treatment). Since there may be strong links between the prognosis of patients and the probability that they will be offered and accept a treatment (sometimes called 'confounding'), the analyses of these cohort analytic studies are difficult and often involve trying to correct for known confounders (such as disease severity) by statistical methods (all the way from simply comparing outcomes within patients with different degrees of severity to quite fancy multivariate analyses). But we can't adjust for what we don't yet know about the determinants of disease outcomes, so you have to be cautious in interpreting cohort studies.

107

And for rare or late complications of treatments, not even cohort studies are big enough and often you'll have to rely on studies conducted vertically in Table 3a4.2 by assembling cases (**a+c**) who already have the bad outcome, assembling a second group of 'controls' (**b+d**) who don't have the bad outcome and tracking back in their histories or records to determine the proportions of each group who were exposed to the suspect treatment (**a** or **b**): a case-control study. This is, in fact, what was done in trying to sort out the fenoterol problem: asthma deaths (cases) were compared with living asthma patients (controls) for their use of fenoterol and these comparisons were 'adjusted' for the severity of their asthma. The problem of confounding (of prognosis with exposure) is even worse in case-control studies than in cohort studies, for often it is impossible to measure the confounders among cases, even if they are known.* For this reason, case-control studies are viewed with even greater caution than cohort studies. Finally, you may find reports of one or a few patients who developed the bad outcome while under treatment (just cell **a**). If the outcome is unique and dramatic (phocomelia in children born to women who took thalidomide) case reports and case series may be enough, but usually they simply point to the need for the other types of studies.

As with other issues in clinical and health care, the best evidence on adverse effects will come from a systematic review of all the relevant studies and these should always be your primary targets when searching for the best external evidence. Systematic reviews of randomized trials or cohort studies may possess sufficiently large numbers of patients to identify even rare adverse effects. Whether appraising a systematic review or an individual study, you'll need to take into account how it assembled and assessed its members and now that you've learned how to recognize the sort of study you're reading, you can apply the guides in Table 3a4.1:

1. From the foregoing discussion, it's clear why you want the report to describe clearly defined groups of

---

* Dead patients tell no tales and information about exposures to lethal treatments may perish with their victims.

108

patients, similar in all important ways other than exposure to the treatment (to get rid of confounders).

2. Moreover, it makes sense that you should place greater confidence in reports of studies in which treatment exposures and clinical outcomes were measured the same ways in both groups (you'd not want one group studied more exhaustively than the other, because this would lead to reporting a greater occurrence of exposure or outcome in the more intensively studied group).

3. Furthermore, in a report concluding that the treatment was innocent, you'd want the follow-up of study patients to have been complete and long enough for the bad effects to have had time to reveal themselves.

4. Finally, you'd want to determine whether the association met at least some common-sense 'diagnostic tests for causation':

• you'd want to be sure that the exposure (say, use of a psychotropic drug) preceded the onset of the bad outcome (say, behavior ending in suicide), and wasn't just a 'marker' (say, of depression) that it was already underway;

• the validity of a claim that a treatment causes an adverse outcome receives a real boost when increasing doses or durations of the treatment are associated with increasing frequency or severity of the adverse outcome: a 'dose-response' effect;

• the validity of a claim is also boosted if there is documentation that the adverse effect decreased or disappeared when the treatment was withdrawn ('dechallenge') and worsened or reappeared when the treatment was reintroduced ('rechallenge');

• if you are fortunate enough to have found a systematic review of the question, you can determine whether the association of exposure to the suspect treatment and the adverse outcome is consistent from study to study. When it is, your confidence in the validity of the association deserves to increase;

• finally, it boosts your confidence when the association makes biological sense.

109

Evidence-based Medicine

If the report fails to meet the first three minimum standards, you're better off abandoning it and continuing your search. On the other hand, if you're satisfied that the report meets these minimum guides, you can decide whether the relation between exposure and outcome is strong and convincing enough for you to need to do something about it and that's discussed in Section 3b4.

Further reading

Levine M, Walter S D, Lee H, Haines T, Holbrook A, Moyer V for the Evidence-Based Medicine Working Group. Users' guides to the medical literature: IV. How to use an article about harm. JAMA 1994; 271: 1615–19.

Section 3b1

Is this evidence about a diagnostic test important?

In deciding whether the evidence about a diagnostic test is important, we will focus on a modern way of thinking about diagnosis that takes into account both components of evidence-based medicine: your individual clinical expertise and the best external evidence. The former is your prior assessment of diagnostic possibilities before you do the test ('prior or pretest probabilities') and the latter is the ability of the test to distinguish patients with and without the target disorder (both the oldfashioned concepts of sensitivity and specificity and the newfangled and more powerful ideas around likelihood ratios). We'll show you how to combine these two elements of EBM to refine your estimates of the target disorder ('posterior or post-test probabilities') and make the diagnosis. Diagnostic tests that produce big changes from pretest to post-test probabilities are important and likely to be useful to you in your practice.

Where do these pretest probabilities come from? Usually they are derived from your own accumulating clinical experience, specific for the setting in which you work and the sorts of patients you see. As a result, pretest probabilities for the same target disorder can vary widely between and within countries and between primary, secondary and tertiary care. We have summarized some published pretest probabilities in Table 3b1.1 and more are available from our Website.

Suppose that you're working up a patient with anemia and think that the probability that they have iron deficiency anemia is 50%; that is, the odds are about 50–50 so that it's due to iron deficiency. When you present the patient to your boss, you ask for an educational prescription to determine the usefulness of performing a serum ferritin on your patient as a means of detecting iron deficiency anemia. Suppose further that, in filling your prescription, you find a systematic

---

Table 3b1.1 Some pretest probabilities

Patient problem	Clinical setting	Target disorder	Pretest probability
Melena in a 50-year-old man who drinks 25 units of alcohol a week but has no stigmata of liver disease	Emergency room in North America	Varices	5%
		Benign ulcer	55%
		Gastritis	40%
Symptomless 60-69-year-olds	Primary care	Undiagnosed colon cancer: all patients	0.5%
		positive family history	1.5%
Symptomless	Primary care	≥ 75% stenosis of one or more coronary arteries	
Woman 30–39 y/o			0.3%
60–69 y/o			6%
Man 30–39 y/o			2%
60–69 y/o			12%
Non-anginal chest pain			
Woman 30–39 y/o			1%
60–69 y/o			19%
Man 30–39 y/o			5%
60–69 y/o			28%
Atypical angina			
Woman 30–39 y/o			4%
60–69 y/o			54%
Man 30–39 y/o			22%
60–69 y/o			67%
Typical angina pectoris			
Woman 30–39 y/o			26%
60–69 y/o			91%
Man 30–39 y/o			70%
60–69 y/o			94%
Symptomless 50 y/o with a solitary pulmonary nodule	Primary care	Cancer for any nodules	50%
		For 3 cm nodules	65%

To find more examples, and to nominate additions to the databank of pretest probabilities, refer to this textbook's Website at: http://cebm.jr2.ox.ac.uk/

review of several studies of this diagnostic test (evaluated against the reference standard of a bone marrow stain for iron), decide that it is valid (based on the guides in Tables 3a3.2 and 3a1.1), and find their results as shown in Table 3b1.2. By the time you've tracked down and studied the external evidence, your patient's serum ferritin comes back at 60 mmol/L. How should you put all this together?

As you can see from Table 3b1.2, your patient's result places them in the top row of the table, either in cell **a** or cell **b**. From that fact you would conclude several things: first, you'd note that 90% of patients with iron deficiency have serum ferritins in the same range as your patient, (a/(a+c), and that property, the proportion of patients with the target disorder who have positive test results, is called sensitivity.

Table 3b1.2 Results of a systematic review of serum ferritin as a diagnostic test for iron deficiency anemia

		Target disorder (iron deficiency anemia)		Totals
		Present	Absent	
Diagnostic test result (serum ferritin)	Positive (<65 mmol/L)	a 731	b 270	a+b 1001
	Negative (≥65 mmol/L)	c 78	d 1500	c+d 1578
	Totals	a+c 809	b+d 1770	a+b+c+d 2579

Sensitivity = **a**/(**a**+**c**) = 731/809 = 90%
Specificity = **d**/(**b**+**d**) = 1500/1770 = 85%
LR+ = sens/(1−spec) = 90%/15% = 6
LR− = (1−sens)/spec = 10%/85% = 0.12
Positive predictive value = **a**/(**a**+**b**) = 731/1001 = 73%
Negative predictive value = **d**/(**c**+**d**) = 1500/1578 = 95%
Prevalence = (**a**+**c**)/(**a**+**b**+**c**+**d**) = 809/2579 = 32%
Pretest odds = prevalence/(1−prevalence) = 31%/69% = 0.45
Post-test odds = pretest odds × likelihood ratio
Post-test probability = post-test odds/(post-test odds +1)

And you might also note that only 15% of patients with other causes for their anemia have results in the same range as your patient,* which means that your patient's result would be about six times as likely (90% / 15%) to be seen in someone with, as opposed to someone without, iron deficiency anemia and that's called the likelihood ratio for a positive test result. Furthermore, since you thought ahead of time (before you had the result of the serum ferritin) that your patient's odds of iron deficiency were 50–50, that's called a pretest odds of 1:1 and, as you can see from the formulae towards the bottom of Table 3b1.2, you can multiply that pretest odds of 1 by the likelihood ratio of 6 to get the post-test odds of iron deficiency anemia after the test: 1×6 = 6. Since, like most clinicians, you may be more comfortable thinking in terms of probabilities than odds, this post-test odds of 6:1 converts (as you can see at the bottom of Table 3b1.2) to a post-test probability of 6/(6+1) = 6/7 = 86%. So it looks like you've made the diagnosis and this diagnostic test looks worthwhile.

(To check yourself out on these calculations, try the same ferritin result for a patient who, like those in the table, has a pretest odds of 0.47;‡ you'll know you did it right if you wind up with an answer identical to its equivalent, the positive predictive value.)

Extremely high values of sensitivity and specificity are useful, but not for the reasons you may think.‡ When a test has a very high sensitivity (such as the loss of retinal vein pulsation in increased intracranial pressure), a negative result (the presence of pulsation) effectively rules out the diagnosis (of raised intracranial pressure) and one of our clinical clerks suggested that we apply the mnemonic SnNout to such findings (when a sign has a high Sensitivity, a Negative result

---

* The complement of this proportion is called specificity and it describes the proportion of patients who do not have the target disorder who have negative or normal test results, **d**/(b+**d**).

‡ The post-test odds are 0.45 × 6 = 2.7 and the post-test probability is 2.7/3.7 = 73%. Note that this is identical to the positive predictive value.

‡ On first encounter, most learners think that tests with high sensitivity rule in diagnoses and tests with high specificity rule them out; the reverse is the case.

rules *out* the diagnosis). Similarly, when a sign has a very high specificity (such as a fluid wave for ascites), a positive result effectively rules in the diagnosis (of ascites); not surprisingly, our clinical clerks call such a finding a SpPin (when a sign has a high *Specificity*, a *Positive* result rules *in* the diagnosis). We've listed some SpPins and SnNouts in Table 3b1.3 and have generated a longer list on our Website.

Although the serum ferritin determination looks impressive when viewed in terms of its sensitivity (90%) and specificity (85%), the newer way of expressing its accuracy with likelihood ratios reveals its even greater power and, in this particular example, shows how we can be misled by the fact that the old sensitivity–specificity approach restricts us to just two levels (positive and negative) of the test result. Most test results, like serum ferritin, can be divided into several levels and in Table 3b1.4 we show you a particularly useful way of dividing test results into five levels. When this is done, one extreme level of the test result can be shown to rule in the diagnosis and in this case you can SpPin 59% of the patients with iron deficiency anemia, despite the unimpressive sensitivity (59%) that would have been achieved if the ferritin results had been split at this level. Likelihood ratios of 10 or more, when applied to pretest probabilities of 33% or more (.33/.67 = pretest odds of 0.5) will generate post-test probabilities of 5/6 = 83% or more. Moreover, the other extreme level can SnNout 75% of those who do not have iron deficiency anemia (again despite a not very impressive specificity (59%)). Likelihood ratios of 0.1 or less, when applied to pretest probabilities of 33% or less (.33/.67 = pretest odds of 0.5) will generate post-test probabilities of 0.05/1.05 = 5% or less. Two other intermediate levels can move a 50% prior probability (pretest odds of 1:1) to the useful but not usually diagnostic post-test probabilities of 4.8/5.8 = 83% and 0.39/1.39 = 28%. And one indeterminate level in the middle (containing about 10% of both sorts of patients) can be seen to be uninformative, with a likelihood ratio of 1. We've shown the effects of these sorts of likelihood ratios on these sorts of pretest probabilities in Table 3b1.5.

Table 3b1.3 Some SpPins and SnNouts

Target disorder	SpPin (& specificity) [presence rules in the target disorder]	SnNout (& sensitivity) [absence rules out the target disorder]
Ascites (by imaging or tap)*	Fluid wave (92%)	History of ankle swelling (93%)
Pleural effusion†	Auscultatory percussion note loud and sharp (100%)	Auscultatory percussion note soft and/or dull (96%)
Increased intracranial pressure (by CAT scan or direct measurement)‡	Loss of spontaneous retinal vein pulsation (100%)	
Cancer as a cause of lower back pain (by further investigation)§		Age >50 or cancer history or unexplained weight loss or failure of conservative therapy (100%)
Sinusitis (by further investigation)¶	Maxillary toothache or purulent nasal secretion or poor response to nasal decongestants or abnormal transillumination or history of coloured nasal discharge	
Alcohol abuse or dependency**	Yes to ≥3 of the CAGE questions (99.8%)	
Splenomegaly (by imaging)††	Positive percussion (Nixon method) and palpation	
Non-urgent cause for dizziness‡‡	Positive head-hanging test and either vertigo or vomiting (94%)	

To find more examples, and to nominate additions to the databank of SpPins and SnNouts, refer to this textbook's Website at: http://cebm.jr2.ox.ac.uk/

* JAMA 1992; 267: 2645–8.
† J Gen Int Med 1994; 9: 71–4.
‡ Arch Neurol 1978; 35: 37–40.
§ JAMA 1992; 268: 760–5.
• JAMA 1993; 270: 1242–6.
** Amer J Med 1987; 82: 231–5.
†† JAMA 1993; 270: 2218–21.
‡‡ JAMA 1994; 271: 385–8.

Table 3b1.4 The usefulness of five levels of a diagnostic test result

Diagnostic test result	Serum ferritin (mmol/L)	Target disorder present		Target disorder absent		Likelihood ratio	Diagnostic Impact
		Number	%	Number	%		
Very positive	<15	474	59%	20	1.1%	52	Rule in SpPin
Moderately positive	15–34	175	22%	79	4.5%	4.8	Intermediate high
Neutral	35–64	82	10%	171	10%	1	Indeterminate
Moderately negative	65–94	30	3.7%	168	9.5%	0.39	Intermediate low
Extremely negative	≥95	48	5.9%	1332	75%	0.08	Rule out SnNout
		809	100%	1770	100%		

Table 3b1.5 Some post-test probabilities generated by five levels of a diagnostic test result

Likelihood ratio	Post-test probability of the target disorder for different pretest probabilities						Diagnostic Impact
	Pre-test 5%	Pre-test 10%	Pre-test 20%	Pre-test 30%	Pre-test 50%	Pre-test 70%	
Very positive 10	34%	53%	71%	81%	91%	96%	Rule in SpPin
Moderately positive 3	14%	25%	43%	56%	75%	88%	Intermediate high
Neutral 1	5%	10%	20%	30%	50%	70%	Indeterminate
Moderately negative 0.3	1.5%	3.2%	7%	11%	23%	41%	Intermediate low
Extremely negative 0.1	0.5%	1%	2.5%	4%	9%	19%	Rule out SnNout

Finally, there's an easier way of manipulating all these probability↔odds calculations and a nomogram for doing so appears as Figure 3b1.1 and in the pocket cards that come with this book. You can check out your understanding of this nomogram by replicating the results in Table 3b1.5.

To your surprise (we reckon!) your patient's test result generates an indeterminate likelihood ratio of only 1 and the test which you thought might be very useful, based on the sensitivity and specificity way of looking at things, really hasn't been helpful in moving you toward the diagnosis, so you'll have to think about other tests (including perhaps the reference standard of a bone marrow examination) to sort this out.

More and more reports of diagnostic tests are providing multilevel likelihood ratios as measures of their accuracy. When they only report sensitivity and specificity, you can sometimes find a table with more levels and generate your own set of likelihood ratios or you can find a scatter plot (of test results versus diagnoses) that is good enough for you to be able to split into levels. Or, if all you have is sensitivity and specificity, you can generate likelihood ratios from them by reference to the formulae in Table 3b1.2 (the likelihood ratio for a positive test result = LR+ = sensitivity/[1-specificity] and the likelihood ratio for a negative test result = LR− = [1-sensitivity]/specificity).

Some reports into the accuracy of diagnostic tests go beyond even likelihood ratios and one of them deserves mention here. This extension considers multiple diagnostic tests as a cluster or sequence of tests for a given target disorder. These multiple results can be presented in different ways, either as clusters of positive/negative results or as multivariate scores, and in either case they can be ranked and handled just like other multilevel likelihood ratios.

In any event, having decided that a diagnostic test produces important changes from pretest to post-test probabilities, you might want to study the final issue, described in Section 4.1, of how to integrate the results of this critical appraisal with your individual clinical expertise and apply the results to your own patient (but if you jumped to this second step without first determining whether the evidence about this diagnostic test was valid, you'd better go back to Section 3a1 first!).

Further reading

Sackett D L, Haynes R B, Guyatt G H, Tugwell P. Clinical epidemiology: a basic science for clinical medicine, 2nd edn. Little, Brown, Boston, 1991. Chapter 4 (for interpreting diagnostic tests).

Jaeschke R, Guyatt G H, Sackett D L for the Evidence-Based Medicine Working Group. Users' guides to the medical literature. VI. How to use an article about a diagnostic test. A. Are the results of the study valid? JAMA 1994; 271: 389–91. B. What are the results and will they help me in caring for my patients? JAMA 1994; 271: 703–7.

Nomogram for interpreting diagnostic test result

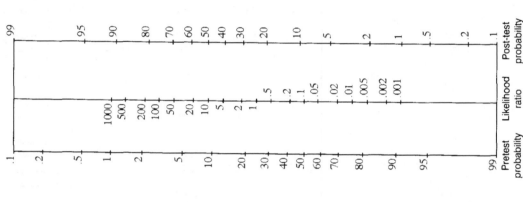
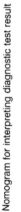

Figure 3b1.1 A likelihood ratio nomogram. Adapted from Fagan T J 1975 Nomogram for Bayes's Theorem (c). New England Journal of Medicine 293: 257

Section 3b2

Is this evidence about prognosis important?

Guides for making this decision appear in Table 3b2.1. First, how likely are the outcomes over time? Diseases usually have more than a single outcome of interest and these can occur in several combinations and at different times following the onset of the disease. Thus, for each important disease outcome, you should examine the article to see how likely each of these outcomes is over time. Typically they are reported as percentage survival at a particular point in time (such as 1-year or 5-year survival rates) and as survival curves of various kinds. Another form of result, common in cancer studies, is the median survival, indicating the length of follow-up by which 50% of the study sample have died. The more numerous the outcome possibilities and the more variable the timing of these outcomes are, the more complex such results can be.

Figure 3b2.1 illustrates some different patterns of prognosis, each leading to different conclusions about prognosis. They are presented in the most frequent format used to describe prognosis, a survival curve that depicts, at each point in time, the proportion (often expressed as a %) of the original study population who have NOT yet had an outcome event.* In panel A, virtually no patients have had events by the end of the study, so either the prognosis is very good (in which case the study is very useful to you) or the study is too short (in which case it's not very useful!). Panels B, C and D depict a serious disease, with only

---

* How such survival curves are constructed is not described in detail in this book, so don't look for it! In brief, it is done by some clever methods that combine the results from patients who have been followed for just short periods of time as well as long ones and who have had outcomes occur early, late or not at all. Often the strategy used here is a 'life table' method, if you want to look it up.

Table 3b2.1 Is this evidence about prognosis important?

1. How likely are the outcomes over time?
2. How precise are the prognostic estimates?

20% of patients surviving at 1 year; you could tell such patients, then, that their chances of surviving for a year are 20%. Note, however, that the shapes of these curves are quite different, so that the median survival (by which time half of them have succumbed) is 9 months for the disorder described in panel B but only 3 months for the disorder described in panel C. The survival pattern is a steady, uniform decline only in panel D and we hope you can see why the best answer to 'How much time have I got, doc?' often is the time at which half the study patients have died (or suffered some other event of interest); this is called the median survival.

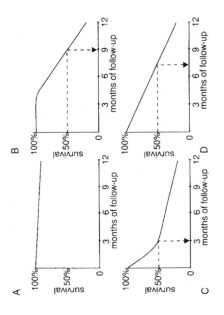

Figure 3b2.1 Prognosis shown as survival curves. Panel A: Good prognosis (or too short a study!). Panel B: Good prognosis early, then worsening, with a median survival of 9 months. Panel C: Bad prognosis early, then better, with a median survival of 3 months. Panel D: Steady prognosis, with a median survival of 6 months

The second guide asks you to consider how precise the prognostic statements are. As we mentioned in Section 3a2, investigators study prognosis in a sample of diseased patients, not in the whole population of everyone who has ever had the disease. Purely by the play of chance, then, the identical study done 100 times over with different samples from that same whole population would yield differing results. In deciding whether these prognostic results are important, then, you will need some means of judging just how much these results could vary by chance alone, that is, the precision of the results. This is best done with the 95% confidence interval:* in those 100 repetitions of the identical study with different samples, 95 would be within a calculable distance of the true prognosis (some lower and some higher). For example, an article on the prognosis of first strokes among 675 patients reported a case-fatality rate of 20% in the first month, with the 95% confidence interval of 17–23%; that interval is pretty narrow and if the report was valid, it looks important as well. If, on the other hand, that 20% was based on just 20 patients, the 95% confidence interval on death in the first month would run from 2% to 38% and that is so wide (almost 20-fold) that you couldn't regard the result as important and potentially useful to you. The text, tables or graphs should tell you the confidence interval for the prognosis and you can decide whether it is too big for you to trust it.

That completes your critical appraisal of evidence about prognosis. If you decide that the evidence you've found is both valid and important, you could go to Section 2 of Chapter 4 (page 164) and decide whether and how to apply it to your patient.

---

* We describe the confidence interval in the Appendix. In this case, the confidence interval on a prognosis (expressed as a decimal) is the observed result plus or minus 1.96 times the square root of {[(the observed result) × (1 – the observed result)] / sample size}. So, for the original study 20% = 0.2 and the confidence interval becomes 0.2 +/– 1.96 times the square root of {[(0.2) × (0.8)]/675} or 0.2 +/– 0.03 or 17–23%. As a check on your understanding, you can see if you can calculate the confidence interval when the sample is just 40 stroke patients.

Further reading

Laupacis A, Wells G, Richardson W S, Tugwell P for the Evidence-Based Medicine Working Group. Users' guides to the medical literature. V. How to use an article about prognosis. JAMA 1994; 272: 234–7.

Section 3b3

Is this evidence about a treatment important?

This section will help you determine the size and potential benefits of the effects of the treatment described in a report, whether you've decided (from the previous section) that the report is valid or whether you start here. Because our primary perspective in this book is the individual clinician, the main measure we will show you how to develop and use is the number of patients a clinician needs to treat in order to prevent one additional adverse outcome (NNT) and along the way we will show you both the absolute risk reduction (ARR) and relative risk reduction (RRR) in the occurrence of adverse outcomes achieved by active therapy. We'll also introduce you to the bare bones of assessing the results of an economic analysis, a more complex method that we employ in determining the effects of therapy when we are taking the broader perspective (usually in collaboration with health managers) of deciding how groups of patients, or society as a whole, should be provided or offered treatments in the way that best uses scarce resources such as hospital beds, drugs, operating time, clinicians and money. Finally, we'll give you a brief description of how evidence on the effects of therapy can be formulated into a clinical decision analysis.

In Section 3 of Chapter 4, we'll show you how to extrapolate the measures from each of these three approaches to individual patients, in order to answer the question: Can I apply these results to my patient?

Is the evidence from this randomized trial important?

Introducing some measures of the effects of therapy

Knowing whether you should be impressed with the results of a valid therapeutic trial requires two steps: first, finding the

most useful clinical expression of these results (or converting data from the report into this most useful expression); and second, comparing those results with the results of other treatments for other conditions. We'll take these one at a time.

The relative risk reduction (RRR)

The Diabetes Control and Complications Trial into the effect of intensive diabetes therapy on the development and progression of neuropathy, which we've summarized in Table 3b3.1, confirmed neuropathy occurred among 9.6% of patients randomized to usual care (1–2 insulin injections/day to prevent glycemic symptoms; we'll call that the control event rate or CER) and 2.8% (we'll call that the experimental event rate or EER) among patients randomized to intensive therapy (insulin pump or =>3 injections per day).

This difference was statistically highly significant, but how might this treatment effect be expressed in terms of its clinical significance? The traditional measure of this effect is the proportional or 'relative' risk reduction (abbreviated RRR in our journal), calculated as (CER–EER)/CER. In this example, the RRR is (9.6% – 2.8%) / 9.6% or 71%; intensive therapy reduced the risk of developing neuropathy by 71%.

Why not confine our description of the clinical significance of this result to the relative risk reduction (RRR)? The reason is that the RRR fails to discriminate huge absolute treatment effects (10 times those observed in this trial) from trivial ones (one ten-thousandth of those observed here). For example, if the rates of neuropathy were 10 times those observed in this trial (the 'high hypothetical case' in Table 3b3.1), and a whopping 96% of control patients and 28% of intensively treated patients developed neuropathy, the relative risk reduction would remain unchanged: RRR = (96% – 28%) / 96% or 71%. And if a trivial 0.00096% of control and 0.00028% of intensively treated patients developed neuropathy (the 'low hypothetical case' in Table 3b3.1), the

Table 3b3.1 Clinically useful measures of the effects of treatment

The occurrence of neuropathy	Event rates (diabetic neuropathy)		Relative risk reduction RRR = CER−EER / CER	Absolute risk reduction ARR = (CER−EER)	Number needed to be treated (to prevent one event) NNT = 1/ARR
	Usual insulin regimen (CER)	Intensive insulin regimen (EER)			
In the actual trial	9.6%	2.8%	$\frac{9.6\% - 2.8\%}{9.6\%}$ = 71%	9.6% − 2.8% = 6.8%	$\frac{1}{6.8\%}$ = 14.7 or 15
High hypothetical case A	96%	28%	$\frac{96\% - 28\%}{96\%}$ = 71%	96% − 28% = 68%	$\frac{1}{68\%}$ = 1.47 or 2
Low hypothetical case B	0.00096%	0.00028%	$\frac{(0.00096\% - 0.00028\%)}{0.00096\%}$ = 71%	0.00096% − 0.00028% = 0.00068%	$\frac{1}{0.00068\%}$ = 147 000

relative risk reduction is as before: RRR still = (0.00096% − 0.00028%) / 0.00096 = 71%! This is because the relative risk reduction discards the underlying susceptibility (or 'baseline risk') of patients entering randomized trials; as a result, the relative risk reduction cannot discriminate huge risks and benefits from small ones.

The absolute risk reduction (ARR)

In contrast to these non-discriminating relative risk reductions, the absolute difference in the rates of neuropathy between control and experimental patients (CER−EER) clearly does discriminate between these extremes and this measure is called the absolute risk reduction or ARR. In the trial, the ARR or (CER−EER) = 9.6% − 2.8% = 6.8%; in the high hypothetical case, where 96% of control patients and 28% of intensively treated patients developed neuropathy, the ARR = 96% − 28% = 68% and in the low hypothetical case in which a trivial 0.00096% of control and 0.00028% of intensively treated patients developed neuropathy, the ARR = 0.00096% − 0.00028% = 0.00068%. These absolute risk reductions retain the underlying susceptibility of patients and provide more complete information than relative risk reductions. And when treatment increases the occurrence of some good event (rather than decreasing the occurrence of some bad event) we can generate an absolute risk increase or ARI. But, unlike relative risk reductions (RRRs), absolute risk reductions and increases (ARRs and ARIs) are difficult to remember and don't slip easily off the tongue at the bedside (lots of clinicians become queasy with numbers less than 1.0).

The number of patients that need to be treated (NNT) to prevent one bad outcome

If, however, we divide the absolute risk reduction into 1 (that is, if we 'invert' the ARR or 'take its reciprocal' so that it becomes 1/ARR), we generate a very useful number, for it represents the number of patients we need to treat (NNT)

with the experimental therapy in order to prevent one of them from developing the bad outcome.* In this case, we would generate the number of diabetics we would need to treat with the intensive regimen in order to prevent one of them from developing neuropathy. In the trial, the NNT is 1/ARR or 1/6.8% or 14.7; we usually round that number upwards (in this case, to 15) and we now can say that for every 15 patients who are treated with the more intensive insulin regimen, one will be prevented from developing diabetic neuropathy.

Is this a large or a small number of patients that need to be treated to prevent one bad outcome? Now we're ready to pursue that second step in deciding whether to be impressed with the valid results of a therapeutic trial. Like many important matters in medicine, the answer has to do with clinical significance, not statistical significance. This NNT of 15 certainly is far smaller than the number of patients we'd need to treat in the extremely low hypothetical example, in which 1/ARR becomes 1/(0.00068%) or an NNT of more than 147 000, a figure so vast that we can't imagine anyone judging that it was worth the effort. We can get a better idea by comparing this NNT of 15 with that for other interventions we are familiar with in medicine.

In doing so, we add the additional dimension of the duration of therapy: in the diabetes trial treatment went on for an average of 6.5 years, meaning that we need to treat about 15 diabetics for about 6.5 years with an intensive insulin regimen to prevent one of them from developing neuropathy. How does this compare with other treatments, over other durations, for other conditions? We show some of them (with the event rates appearing as decimals rather than percents) in Table 3b3.2. Beginning on an optimistic note, we need to treat only about 20 chest pain patients who appear to be having heart attacks with streptokinase and aspirin to save a life at 5 weeks. On the other hand, we need to treat about 70 elderly hypertensives for 5 years with antihypertensive drugs

---

* Similarly, 1/ARI tells us how many individuals we need to treat to cause one additional good outcome.

to save one life, about 100 men with no evidence of coronary heart disease for 5 years with aspirin to prevent one heart attack and about 10 patients with symptomatic moderate to severe carotid artery stenosis with endarterectomy to prevent one major or fatal stroke over the following 2 years.

We think that the 'number needed to be treated' (NNT) to prevent one event is the most useful measure of the clinical effort we and our patients must expend in order to help them avoid bad outcomes to their illnesses. Note, however, that this is a measure with real meaning for clinicians, but not for individual patients (who are interested in Ns of 1, not NNTs). Furthermore, because we are focusing here on the magnitude of the treatment effect, rather than on the probability that we have drawn a false-positive conclusion that the treatment is at all effective (when it is not), we should employ confidence intervals around the NNT, specifying the 'limits' within which we can confidently state the true NNT lies (95% of the time), rather than focus just on p-values. Readers who want to brush up on confidence intervals can refer to the Appendix.

Since we are interested in the risks as well as the benefits of treatments, we can generate a parallel 'number needed to harm' or NNH to express the downside of therapy. For example, if anticoagulation carries an annual risk of major bleeding of 2%, the NNH is 1/2% = 50.

Overviews and metaanalyses often provide NNTs, but sometimes only report odds ratios. The latter are not the same as RRRs and can be converted into RRRs only when you know the patient's expected event rate (PEER) by using the formula:

$$NNT = \frac{1 - [PEER \times (1 - OR)]}{(1 - PEER) \times PEER \times (1 - OR)}$$

To help you 'translate' odds ratios to NNTs (without having to crank through this formula), we've summarized several of them in Table 3b3.3.

The NNT from the published report, in light of your own clinical expertise and compared with those in Table 3b3.2, will give you an idea of whether the treatment is potentially

¶¶ Am J Obstet Gynecol 1995;173:322-35. EBM 1996;1:92.
§§ N Engl J Med 1991;325:445-53.
‡‡ Lancet 1993;341:973-8.
†† Lancet 1995;345:1455-63. EBM 1996;1:44.
** N Engl J Med 1995;333:1184-9. EBM 1996;1:87.
¶ BMJ 1985;291:97-104.
§ JAMA 1967;202:116-22
‡ Lancet 1988;2:349-60.
† Diabetes Res Clin Pract 1995;28:103-17
* Ann Intern Med 1995;122:561-8. EBM 1995:1:9.

To find more examples, and to nominate additions to the databank of NNTs, refer to this textbook's Web Page at: http://cebm.jr2.ox.ac.uk/

Table 3b3.2 Some NNTs for different treatments

Condition or disorder	Intervention	Events being prevented	Control Event Rate CER	Experimental Event Rate EER	Duration of follow-up	NNT to prevent one additional event
Diabetes (IDDM)*	Intensive insulin regimens	Diabetic neuropathy	0.096	0.028	6.5 years	15
Diabetes (NIDDM)†	Intensive insulin regimens	Worse diabetic retinopathy	0.38	0.13	6 years	4
		Nephropathy	0.30	0.10		5
Acute myocardial infarction‡	Streptokinase and Aspirin	Death at 5 weeks	0.134	0.081	5 weeks	19
		Death at 2 years	0.216	0.174	2 years	24
Diastolic blood pressure 115-129 mm Hg§	Antihypertensive drugs	Death, stroke or myocardial infarction	0.1286	0.0137	1.5 years	3
Diastolic blood pressure 90-109 mm Hg¶	Antihypertensive drugs	Death, stroke or myocardial infarction	0.0545	0.0467	5.5 years	128
Independent elderly people**	Comprehensive geriatric home assessment	Long-term nursing home admission	0.10	0.04	3 years	17
Pregnant women with eclampsia††	iv MgSO₄ (vs. diazepam)	Recurrent convulsion	0.279	0.132	hours	7
Healthy women ages 50-69‡‡	Breast examination plus mammography	Death from breast cancer	0.00345	0.00252	9 years	1075
Symptomatic high-grade carotid artery stenosis§§	Carotid endarterectomy	Major stroke or death	0.181	0.08	2 years	10
Preterm babies¶¶	Antenatal corticosteroids	Respiratory distress syndrome	0.23	0.13	days	11

Table 3b3.3 Translating odds ratios to NNTs

Patient's expected event rate (PEER)	Odds ratio				
	0.9	0.8	0.7	0.6	0.5
.05	209*	104	69	52	41†
.10	110	54	36	27	21
.20	61	30	20	14	11
.30	46	22	14	10	8
.40	40	19	12	9	7
.50	38	18	11	8	6
.70	44	20	13	9	6
.90	101‡	46	27	18	12§

The numbers in the body of the table are the NNTs for the corresponding odds ratios at that particular patient's expected event rate (PEER).
* The relative risk reduction (RRR) here is 49%.
† The RRR here is 10%.
‡ The RRR here is 1%.
§ The RRR here is 9%.

useful for your patient. In the next chapter, we will show you a very simple way to find out whether this potential is met for your individual patient.

Section 3b4

Is this evidence about harm important?

The main measure that indicates whether valid evidence that a treatment harms some patients is also impressive (and potentially useful clinically) is the strength of the association between receiving the treatment and suffering the adverse effect. Strength here means the risk or odds of the adverse effect with, as opposed to without, exposure to the treatment; the higher the risk or odds, the greater the strength and the more you should be impressed with it.

Different tactics for estimating the strength of association are used in different types of studies and these are shown in Table 3b4.1. In the randomized trial and cohort study, patients who were and were not exposed to the treatment are carefully followed up to find out whether they develop the adverse outcome, with the risk in the treated patients, relative to untreated patients, calculated as $[a/(a+b)]/[c/(c+d)]$. Thus, if 1000 patients receive a treatment and 20 of them have an adverse outcome, $a=20$ and $a/(a+b) = 20/1000 = 2\%$; and if just two of 1000 patients with the same condition but receiving a different treatment suffered this adverse outcome, $c=2$ and $c/(c+d) = 2/1000 = 0.2\%$ and the relative risk = 2%/0.2% or 10. That is, patients receiving the suspect treatment were 10 times as likely to suffer the adverse outcome as patients treated some other way.

In a case-control study, where patients with and without the adverse outcome are selected and tracked backward to their prior treatments, strength (which in this case is called the odds ratio) can only be indirectly estimated as **ad/bc**. For example, if 100 cases of the adverse outcome are assembled and it is discovered that 90 of them had received the suspect treatment, $a=90$ and $c=10$; if 100 control patients, free of the adverse outcome, are also assembled and it is discovered that only 45 of them received the suspect treatment, **b=45** and **d=55**, and the relative odds = **ad/bc** = (90×55)/(45×10) = 11. That is, patients receiving the suspect treatment are 11 times as likely to suffer the adverse event as patients treated some other way.

How big should relative risks and relative odds become before you should be impressed with them? This question has two answers. First, you'd like to be confident that the relative risk (RR) or relative odds (RO) is really greater than 1 (when RR or RO = 1, the adverse outcome is no greater with than without exposure to the suspect treatment). So, as before, you'd want to be sure that the entire confidence interval remains within a clinically important range of RR or RO. Second, the size of the 'impressive' RR or RO depends on the type of study from which it is generated. Because of the biases we described in case-control studies, you'd want to be sure that the RO was greater than that which could arise from bias alone and you might not want to become impressed with their ROs until they reach 4 or more (some of our colleagues would relax these guides for a serious adverse effect and set them even higher for a trivial one). Since cohort studies are less subject to bias, you might be impressed with RRs of 3 or

Table 3b4.1 Different ways of calculating the strength of an association between a treatment and subsequent adverse outcomes

		Adverse outcome		Totals
		Present (Case)	Absent (Control)	
Exposed to the treatment	Yes (Cohort)	a	b	a+b
	No (Cohort)	c	d	c+d
	Totals	a+c	b+d	a+b+c+d

In a randomized trial or cohort study: relative risk = RR = $[a/(a+b)]/[c/(c+d)]$
In a case-control study: relative odds = RO = **ad/bc**

Table 4.1.1 Questions to answer in applying a valid diagnostic test to an individual patient

1. Is the diagnostic test available, affordable, accurate and precise in your setting?
2. Can you generate a clinically sensible estimate of your patient's pretest probability:
   ● from practice data?
   ● from personal experience?
   ● from the report itself?
   ● from clinical speculation?
3. Will the resulting post-test probabilities affect your management and help your patient?
   ● Could it move you across a test–treatment threshold?
   ● Would your patient be a willing partner in carrying it out?
   ● Would the consequences of the test help your patient reach their goals in all this?

Section 4.1

Can you apply this valid, important evidence about a diagnostic test in caring for your patient?

Having found a valid systematic review or individual report about a diagnostic test and decided that its accuracy is sufficiently high to be useful, how do you integrate it with your individual clinical expertise and apply it to your patient?

There are three questions whose answers dictate this determination, summarized in Table 4.1.1. First, is the diagnostic test available, affordable, accurate and precise in your setting? You obviously can't order a test that's not available but even if it is, you may want to check around to be sure that it's performed and interpreted in a competent, reproducible fashion and that its potential consequences (see below) justify its cost. Moreover, diagnostic tests often behave differently among different subsets of patients, generating higher likelihood ratios in later stages of florid disease and lower likelihood ratios in early, mild stages. This is another reason why multilevel likelihood ratios are helpful, as there are at least theoretical reasons why they should suffer less distortion from this cause. Finally, it is known that at least some diagnostic tests based on symptoms or signs lose power as patients move from primary care to secondary and tertiary care. Reference back to Table 3b1.1 can show you why: if patients are referred onward in part because of symptoms, their primary care clinicians will be sending along patients in both cells **a** and **b** and subsequent evaluations of the accuracy of their symptoms will tend to show falling specificity due to the referral of patients with false-positive findings. If you think that any of these factors may be clinically sensible variations in the likelihood ratios for your test result and see whether the results alter your post-test probabilities in a way that changes your diagnosis (the short-hand term for this sort of exploration is 'sensitivity analysis').

The second question you need to answer is whether you can generate a clinically sensible estimate of your patient's pretest probability. Sometimes you've actually got the data on pretest probabilities from your practice or institution. That's wonderful when it exists and constitutes a reason to consider keeping some records on the pretest probabilities for important diagnoses you eventually make for the specific presenting complaints in which you'd consider this sort of diagnostic test. Sometimes, you've had enough experience both to be able to make this estimation based on your own experience and to know how your estimate can be distorted by your last case (either way, depending on whether you ruled in or ruled out the diagnosis), your most dramatic or embarrassing case (usually this either distorts your pretest odds upwards or makes you reluctant to quit testing until the post-test odds are vanishingly small) or by whether you are an expert in the evaluation or care of patients with this diagnosis (which usually makes you reluctant to miss one).

Early in your career or when you haven't previously encountered this diagnostic situation, you'll be less certain about your patient's pretest probability. When that happens, you can try one or more of the following. First, if

more in them. And because randomized trials are relatively free of bias, any RR whose confidence interval excludes 1 is impressive and warrants further consideration.

Having decided that you are impressed with both the validity and the strength of the relationship between the suspect treatment and the adverse outcome, you then need to translate this into some measure of the impact of changing your treatment strategy on the occurrence of the adverse outcome and decide whether it is worth the effort required to achieve it. The measures we've employed up to now, the RR and OR, don't provide this information very well and you need to return to the concept of the NNT. In this case you are concerned about a bad outcome and you might want to revise the term to the 'number of patients needed to be treated to produce one episode of harm' or NNH. Our reason for doing this is that the RR and OR are fine for telling us whether the link to harm was true, but don't tell us whether the link was clinically important. For example, a cohort study showed that NSAIDs can cause gastrointestinal bleeding and the confidence interval on the relative risk for this adverse outcome included 2. A randomized trial showed that the antiarrhythmic drugs encainide and flecainide can cause death and the confidence interval on the relative risk for this adverse outcome also included 2. But the absolute increase in the risk of bleeding in the former study was small, at about 0.05%, which translates to an NNH of 2000 to cause one more GI bleed, whereas the absolute increase in the risk of death in the latter trial was 4.7% or an NNH of 21 to cause one additional death! Clearly, similar RRs or ORs can lead to very different NNHs and you need the latter as well as the former to make your clinical decision about your patient.

That final step of integrating this external evidence with your clinical expertise is discussed in Section 4.4.

Further reading

Levine M. Walter S D. Lee H. Haines T, Holbrook A. Moyer V for the Evidence-Based Medicine Working Group. Users' guides to the medical literature. IV. How to use an article about harm. JAMA 1994; 271: 1615–19.

Evidence-based Medicine

your setting and patient closely resemble those that appeared in the report, you can use its pretest probability. Or if your patient is a bit different from those in the study, you can use its pretest probability as a starting point and again set off on a sensitivity analysis using clinically sensible variations in pretest probabilities and determining their impact on the test's usefulness. As before, the issue here is not whether your patient is exactly like those in the report, but whether they are so different that the report is of no help in making the diagnosis. Finally, you may simply go straight to a sensitivity analysis in which you plug the likelihood ratios from your report into a range of sensible pretest probabilities and see what the likely range of post-test probabilities will be (perhaps using the entries in Table 3b1.4 on page 124 to help you).

The final question you need to answer is: Will the resulting post-test probabilities affect your management and help your patient? The elements of this answer are three. First, could its results move you across some threshold that would cause you to stop all further testing? Two thresholds should be borne in mind. If the diagnostic test was negative or generated a likelihood ratio well below 1.0, the post-test probability might become so low that you would abandon the diagnosis it was pursuing and turn to other diagnostic possibilities. Put in terms of thresholds, this negative test result has moved you from above to below the 'test threshold' and you won't do any more tests for that diagnostic possibility. On the other hand, if the diagnostic test came back positive or generated a high likelihood ratio, the post-test probability might become so high that you would also abandon further testing because you'd made your diagnosis and would now move to choosing the most appropriate therapy: in these terms, you've now crossed from below to above the 'treatment threshold'. It's only if your diagnostic test result leaves you stranded between the test and treatment thresholds that you'd continue to pursue that initial diagnosis by performing other tests. Although there are some very fancy ways of calculating test and treatment thresholds from test accuracy and the risks and benefits of correct and incorrect

diagnostic conclusions,* intuitive test–treatment thresholds are commonly used by experienced clinicians and are another example of individual clinical expertise.

You may not cross a test–treatment threshold until you've performed several different diagnostic tests and here is where another nice property of the likelihood ratio comes into play. Because the post-test odds for the first diagnostic test you apply are the pretest odds for your second diagnostic test, you needn't switch back and forth between odds and probabilities between tests. You can simply keep multiplying the running product by the likelihood ratio generated from the next test. For example, when a 45-year-old man walks into your office his pretest probability of $\geq 75\%$ stenosis of one or more of his coronary arteries is about 6%. Suppose that he gives you a history of atypical chest pain (only two of the three symptoms of substernal chest discomfort, brought on by exertion, and relieved in <10 minutes by rest: a likelihood ratio of about 13) and that his exercise ECG reveals 2.2 mm of non-sloping ST-segment depression (a likelihood ratio of about 11). Then his post-test probability for coronary stenosis is his pretest probability [converted into odds] times the product of the likelihood ratios generated from his history (13) and exercise ECG (11), with the resulting post-test odds converted back to probabilities (through dividing by its value + 1): $(0.06 / 0.94) \times 13 \times 11 = 9.13 / 10.13 = 90\%$. The final result of these calculations is strictly accurate as long as the diagnostic tests being combined are 'independent' (that is, the probability of a specific result on the second is the same for any result on the first) and we know intuitively that this is not true for most of the diagnostic tests we apply in sequences aiming toward a single diagnosis. Accordingly, we'd want the calculated post-test probability at the end of this sequence to be comfortably above our treatment threshold before we would act upon it. This additional example of how likelihood ratios make lots of implicit diagnostic reasoning explicit is another argument in favor of generating overall

---

* See the recommendations for further reading or N Engl J Med 1980; 302: 1109.

likelihood ratios for sequences or clusters of diagnostic tests, as suggested back in Section 3b1.

We hope that you involved your patient as you worked your way through all the foregoing considerations that lead you to think that the diagnostic test is worth considering. If you haven't, you certainly need to do so now. Every diagnostic test involves some invasion of privacy and some are embarrassing, painful or dangerous. You'll have to be sure that the patient is an informed, willing partner in the undertaking.

Finally, the ultimate question to ask about using any diagnostic test is whether its consequences (reassurance when negative, labeling and possibly generating awful diagnostic and prognostic news if positive, leading to further diagnostic tests and treatments, etc.) will help your patient achieve their goals of therapy. Included here are considerations of how subsequent interventions match clinical guidelines or restrictions on access to therapy designed to optimize the use of finite resources for all members of your society.

Further reading

Jaeschke R. Guyatt G H. Sackett D L for the Evidence-Based Medicine Working Group. Users' guides to the medical literature. VI. How to use an article about a diagnostic test. B. What are the results and will they help me in caring for my patients? JAMA 1994; 271: 703–7.

Section 4.2

Can you apply this valid, important evidence about prognosis in caring for your patient?

Having decided that the evidence you tracked down about prognosis is both valid and important, you now can consider how to use it in your clinical practice. Two guides can help you make these judgments; they appear in Table 4.2.1 and will be considered here.

First, were the study patients sufficiently similar to your own? The first guide asks you to compare your patients to those in the article and since presumably you know your patients well, this means trying to get to know the study patients well enough to compare them. Look for descriptions of the study sample, including the patients' demographics and important clinical characteristics. The more the study patients are like your patients, the more readily you can apply the results to your patients. Inevitably, some differences will turn up, so how similar is similar enough? To help you with this judgment, as in other places in this book, we suggest that you try this question framed the other way: are the study patients so different from yours that you'd expect their outcomes to be so different that they wouldn't be any use to you in making prognostic predictions about your patients?

Second, will this evidence make a clinically important impact on your conclusions about what to offer or tell your patient? If the evidence suggests a good prognosis when patients (especially in the early stages of disease) remain

Table 4.2.1 Can you apply this valid, important evidence about prognosis in caring for your patient?

1. Were the study patients similar to your own?
2. Will this evidence make a clinically important impact on your conclusions about what to offer or tell your patient?

untreated, that could strongly influence your discussion of treatment options with them. If, on the other hand, prognostic information derived from a control group in a randomized trial suggests a gloomy prognosis when no definitive therapy is instituted, your message to your patient would reflect this fact. And even when the prognostic evidence doesn't lead to a treat/don't treat decision, valid evidence is always useful in providing your patient or their family with the information they want to have about what the future is likely to hold for them and their illness.

Further reading

Laupacis A, Wells G, Richardson W S, Tugwell P for the Evidence-Based Medicine Working Group. Users' guides to the medical literature. V. How to use an article about prognosis. JAMA 1994; 272: 234–7.

Section 4.3

Can you apply this valid, important evidence about a treatment in caring for your patient?

In deciding whether valid, potentially useful results apply to your patient, you need once again to integrate the evidence with your clinical expertise. As shown in Table 4.3.1, there are two elements to this integration. The first estimates the impact of the treatment on patients just like yours and the second compares the values and preferences of your patient with the regimen and its consequences.

Estimating the impact of a valid, important treatment result on an individual patient

This element poses two additional questions: Do these results apply to your patient? How great would the potential benefit of therapy actually be for your individual patient?

Do these results apply to your patient?

Your patient wasn't in the trial that established the efficacy of this treatment. Maybe (because of their age, sex, comorbidity, disease severity or for a host of other sociodemographic, biologic or clinical reasons) they wouldn't even have been eligible for the trial. How can you extrapolate* from the external evidence to your individual patient? Rather than slavishly asking: 'Would my patient satisfy the eligibility criteria for the trial?' and rejecting its usefulness if they didn't exactly fit every one of them, we'd suggest bringing in some of your knowledge of human biology and

* Some teachers call this 'generalizing' from the trial, but really it's 'particularizing' to an individual patient, not generalizing to all patients, everywhere. Accordingly, we'll use the more generic term 'extrapolating'.

Table 4.3.1 Are these valid, potentially useful results applicable to your patient?

1. Do these results apply to your patient?
   - Is your patient so different from those in the trial that its results can't help you?
   - How great would the potential benefit of therapy actually be for your individual patient?
2. Are your patient's values and preferences satisfied by the regimen and its consequences?
   - Do your patient and you have a clear assessment of their values and preferences?
   - Are they met by this regimen and its consequences?

clinical experience, turning the question around and asking: 'Is my patient so different from those in the trial that its results cannot help me make my treatment decision?' Pharmacogenetics aside, there are very few situations in which you would expect a drug or diet or operation to produce qualitatively different results in patients inside a trial and those who don't quite fit its eligibility criteria. Only if you conclude that your patient is so different from those in the study that its results simply don't inform your treatment decision should you discard its results.

What about subgroups?

Sometimes treatments appear to benefit some subgroups of patients but not others. For example, some of the early trials of aspirin for transient ischemic attacks suggested that this drug was efficacious in men but not in women. As is usually the case, this 'qualitative' difference in the effects of therapy (helpful for one group but useless or harmful in another) was a chance finding and later trials and overviews confirmed that aspirin is efficacious in women. The results from megatrials and overviews suggest that extrapolations from the overall results of individual trials usually are correct when applied to subgroups of patients in those trials. If you think that you may be dealing with one of the exceptions to this rule and that the treatment you're examining really does work in a qualitatively different way among

Table 4.3.2 Should you believe apparent qualitative differences in the efficacy of therapy in some subgroups of patients?

Only if you can say 'yes' to all of the following:
1. Does it really make biologic and clinical sense?
2. Is the qualitative difference both clinically (beneficial for some but useless or harmful for others) and statistically significant?
3. Was it hypothesized before the study began (rather than the product of dredging the data) and has it been confirmed in other, independent studies?
4. Was it one of just a few subgroup analyses carried out in this study?

different patients, you should apply the guides in Table 4.3.2. In particular, unless this difference in response makes biologic sense, was hypothesized before the trial and has been confirmed in a second, independent trial, we'd suggest that you accept the treatment's overall efficacy as the best estimate of its efficacy in your patient.

So, unless there is some really powerful biologic reason for you to think that the treatment, if accepted by your patient, would be totally ineffectual or act in the opposing direction from the way it acted in patients in the study, we think you have good grounds for extrapolating the *direction* of the effect of the treatment on your patient's illness. Having decided that the direction of the treatment effect is likely to be the same as that observed in the study, you can now turn to considering whether that effect is likely to be great or small.

How great would the potential benefit of therapy be for your individual patient?

The trial report informed you about how the treatment worked in the average patient in the trial. How can you translate this to the probable treatment effect in your individual patient? We suggest that the measure we used to decide whether the treatment was potentially useful, the number of patients you need to treat (NNT) to prevent one bad outcome, is useful here. The trick is to translate the NNT

from the study into an NNT that fits your patient. You can do this the longer, harder (and maybe more accurate*) way or the quick and easy (but maybe less accurate) way.

The long way is to estimate the absolute susceptibility of your individual patient for developing the bad outcome over a period of time equal to the duration of the study. If the study you're using had a placebo or no-treatment group or subgroup with features like your patient, you could use their susceptibility† for this purpose. Another way would be to carry out a literature search to find a paper on the prognosis of patients like yours and use that figure. Either way, you'd take the resulting susceptibility (you could express it as a decimal fraction or a percentage, whichever you're more comfortable using) and multiply it by the RRR from the study. The result is the ARR and you can invert it to get the NNT. For example, if you find a prognosis paper suggesting that the susceptibility of your patient for a bad outcome is about 0.4 (the term we use to describe that susceptibility is the 'patient expected event rate' or PEER, so PEER = 40%) over a period of time equal to the duration of the trial that generated an RRR of 50%. Assuming that this RRR applies regardless of the susceptibility of patients in that trial, the ARR is PEER × RRR = 40% × 50% = 20% and the corresponding NNT is 1/ARR = 1/20% = 5 and you'd need to treat just five patients like yours for that length of time to prevent one event. If you would like to avoid these calculations, you can use the nomogram that appears in Figure 4.3.1. But there is an even easier way to estimate an NNT for patients like yours.

As we stated in the previous chapter, one of the reasons why the NNT is useful when interpreting the results of treatment trials is the ease with which it can be extrapolated to your own practice and to individual patients outside the trials. Through some very simple arithmetic, you can estimate NNTs for specific patients. All you need do is estimate the

---

* We're not being cute here. We all are pretty new at this and really don't know!

† Some people, especially when they use a control group to estimate susceptibility, call it 'baseline risk'.

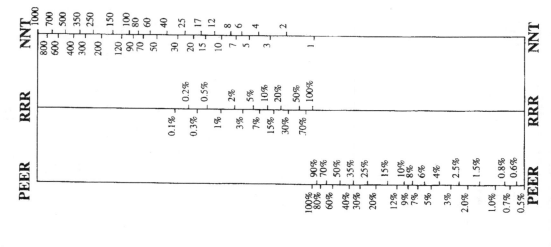

susceptibility of your individual patient (if they were to receive just the control treatment) relative to the average control patient in the reported trial and convert this estimate into a decimal fraction we'll call F (if you judge your patient to be twice as susceptible as those in the trial, F = 2; if your patient is only half as susceptible as the average control patient in the trial, F = 0.5, and if just like the patients in the trial, F = 1). As long as the treatment produces a constant relative risk reduction across the spectrum of susceptibilities,* the NNT for your patient is simply the reported NNT divided by F. Going back to our intensive insulin example in Section 3b3, we learned that a group of clinical investigators had to treat 15 diabetics with intensive insulin regimens for 6.5 years in order to prevent one of them from developing diabetic neuropathy (NNT=15). If you judge that your patient was only half as susceptible as patients in that trial, F = 0.5 and NNT/F = 15/0.5 = 30, so 30 of these less susceptible patients would need to be treated for about 6.5 years with the intensive insulin regimen to prevent one of them from going on to develop neuropathy.

Comparing the values and preferences of your patient with the regimen and its consequences

A return to Table 4.3.1 identifies the steps to be taken here. You and your patient need to achieve a clear assessment of their values and preferences and then determine whether they will be served by the regimen in question. Sometimes the answer will be evident in a few seconds: for a patient having a heart attack, the value of survival and the preference for a simple, low-risk intervention like aspirin, given the efficacy of this regimen, usually makes this decision quickly agreed and acted upon. Other times the answer will take weeks and several visits to sort out: radiation or

adjuvant chemotherapy for stage II carcinoma of the breast or transurethral resection of the prostate for moderate symptoms of prostatism.

* This is a big assumption and we're only beginning to learn when assuming a constant RRR is appropriate (for lots of medical treatments like antihypertensive drugs) and inappropriate (for some operations like carotid endarterectomy, where the RRR rises with increasing susceptibility).

Figure 4.3.1 A nomogram for determining NNTs. Reprinted with permission from Chatellier G et al. The number needed to treat: a clinically useful nomogram in its proper context. BMJ 1996; 312: 426–9.

Section 4.4

Can you apply this valid, important evidence about harm in caring for your patient?

In deciding whether and how to apply valid, potentially important results of a critical appraisal about a harmful treatment to an individual patient, four aspects of individual clinical expertise are important and they are listed in Table 4.4.1.

First, you need to decide whether the results of your critical appraisal can be extrapolated to your patient. As before, the issue is not whether your patient would have met all the inclusion criteria for the systematic review or individual study that demonstrated the harmful effect of the treatment, but whether your patient is so different from those in the report that its results provide no useful guidance for you.

Second, you need to estimate your patient's risk of the adverse outcome relative to the patients in the report. As we described in Section 4.3, if you can express this as a decimal fraction we'll call F (if your patient is twice the risk of those in the report, F=2; if half the risk, F=0.5; if the same risk, F=1) you can then simply divide the number of patients needed to be treated to produce one episode of harm (NNH) from the report by F. If, for example, you decided that a patient you're considering placing on an NSAID is at four times the risk of an upper GI bleed as those in a cohort study

Table 4.4.1 Should these valid, potentially important results of a critical appraisal about a harmful drug change the treatment of an individual patient?

1. Can the study results be extrapolated to this patient?
2. What are this patient's risks of the adverse outcome?
3. What are this patient's preferences, concerns and expectations from this treatment?
4. What alternative treatments are available?

that generated an NNH of 2000, the appropriate NNH for your patient becomes 2000/4 = 500.

Third, as with all clinical decisions, you need to identify and incorporate your patient's preferences, concerns and expectations into your recommendation. If they are 'risk-averse', on the one hand, or willing to gamble side-effects to gain possible treatment benefit, on the other, your discussions of the risks and benefits of the same treatment, even among patients with identical NNHs, may lead to very different treatment plans. At this point you can further modify NNH (or its F, whichever you are more comfortable dealing with) to take into account both your own and your patient's thoughts about the comparative health impacts of the treatment's adverse effect and the clinical event it was being used to prevent in the first place (represented by its NNT). If your patient is risk averse or if either of you thinks that the treatment's adverse effect (e.g. an intracranial bleed from anti-coagulants) is 2–3 times as severe as the event the treatment was intended to prevent (recurrent deep vein thrombosis), you could double or triple the F for the NNH (or cut the NNH by 1/2 or 2/3) and then see how it compares with the NNT. If, on the other hand, your patient is a risk taker or the adverse treatment effect (e.g. cough from an ACE inhibitor) was only 1% as severe as the event the treatment was intended to prevent (death from heart failure), you could reduce the F for the NNH to 0.01 or multiply the NNH by 100.* In either case, the comparison of the treatment's 'adjusted' NNH with its NNT becomes very informative. If a treatment's NNH, after all this adjustment, is lower than its NNT, shouldn't you be considering some therapeutic alternatives? If your time and resources permit, this would be an ideal situation in which to carry out a clinical decision analysis.

Even if the adjusted NNH exceeds the NNT, you still ought to identify the possible alternative treatments (including no treatment!) you could offer your patient instead of the one

* In similar fashion, when a treatment (e.g. NSAIDs for arthritis) causes multiple adverse effects, you would apply a smaller F (or higher NNH) for a minor one (e.g. indigestion) than a major one (e.g. GI hemorrhage).

that produces this adverse effect. If a patient experienced wheezing when their hypertension was treated with a beta-blocker, it is easy to substitute another antihypertensive drug that is free of this side-effect. On the other hand, the alternatives to oral contraceptives for temporary conception control may not be acceptable to your patient, despite the small but real risk of thromboembolism from these drugs.

Further reading

Levine M. Walter S D, Lee H, Haines T, Holbrook A, Moyer V for the Evidence-Based Medicine Working Group. Users' guides to the medical literature. IV. How to use an article about harm. JAMA 1994; 271: 1615–19.

Section 4.6

Teaching methods relevant to the clinical application of the results of critical appraisals to individual patients

In this section we will present some strategies and tactics for teaching learners how to apply the results of their critical appraisals to patients. Because EBM begins and ends with patients, it is natural for us to use patient encounters for closing this loop. The message here is that critical appraisal and other elements of EBM are integral components of the everyday bedside and other clinical discussions of how to diagnose and manage patients and not peripheral topics to be discussed at other places and only when time permits. We will start with some obvious clinical situations, but then move progressively farther afield to demonstrate that closely similar strategies and tactics can be applied to a wide variety of teaching and learning situations. Finally, we will describe how several centers and academic consortia around the world operate 5-day workshops on how to practice EBM.

Working rounds on individual patients

First we will consider the 'working round' in which a clinical team review the problems and progress of patients on a clinical service or in an outpatient setting. These are held in various formats. On an inpatient unit, they might consist of a walking round in which every patient on the service is briefly presented, seen and discussed. In an outpatient setting, they might focus on a single patient who has been asked to stay behind or might consider the entire session's patients after they've left. Finally, they might be quite informal gatherings over coffee in which discussions around patients are tagged onto meetings that deal largely with administrative and housekeeping tasks. When the available time is in harmony with the numbers of patients to be seen

(or at least discussed), these can provide excellent opportunities for teaching and learning EBM. Often, however, time is short and the list of patients long and in those circumstances many services adopt a two-stage approach in which they begin by sitting down and quickly reviewing the patient list and then focus on just those patients in whom major decisions have to be made. In either format, patients are presented (and, if available, examined), followed by discussions in which management decisions are taken and defended with the best available evidence. How might these discussions be organized to maximize the opportunities for learning and practicing EBM? Two tactics are useful here.

The first ties EBM to the presentation of the patient. Back in Chapter 1 we described how the educational prescription could be used to initiate finding and critically appraising evidence and in Table 1.5 we showed how it could form the final element in presenting a new patient. In a similar fashion, as shown in Table 4.6.1, filling that educational Rx can form the final element of presenting a patient already known to the clinical service. In this fashion, the scientific justification for a diagnostic or therapeutic course of action becomes part of describing the past and planning the future care of the patient and serves the decision-making as well as educational requirements of the meeting.

The second tactic concerns the actual presentation of the evidence. The busier the service, the more important that evidence central to management decisions is concisely and quickly presented. This is where the CATs (introduced back in Section 3b7) can come in so handy.* After hearing about and (if possible) examining the patient, the team can gather around the resulting CAT, quickly decide whether its clinical bottom line applies, make the management decision and get on to the next patient (requesting copies of CATs for further study or later use).

---

* For greatest effect, CATs have to be produced in real time while decisions are being made (often easier between visits in ambulatory settings than overnight in inpatient settings). To speed their production, a CAT-Maker is available on disk or via the Website at the Oxford Centre for Evidence-Based Medicine (http://cebm.jr2.ox.ac.uk/).

Table 4.6.1 A guide for learners in presenting an 'OLD'* patient at follow-up rounds

The presentation should summarize 20 things in less than 2 minutes:

1. The patient's surname.
2. Their age.
3. Their gender.
4. Their occupation/social role.
5. When they were admitted.
6. Their chief complaint(s) that led directly to their admission.
7. The number of ACTIVE PROBLEMS that they have at the present time.

And then, for each ACTIVE PROBLEM (a problem could be a symptom, sign, event, diagnosis, injury, psychological state, social predicament, etc.):

8. Its most important symptoms, if any.
9. Its most important signs, if any.
10. The results of diagnostic or other exploratory/confirmatory investigations.
11. The explanation (diagnosis or state) for the problem.
12. The treatment plan instituted for the problem.
13. The response to this treatment plan.
14. The future plans for managing this problem. Repeat 8–14 for each ACTIVE PROBLEM.
15. Your plans for discharge, posthospital care and follow-up.
16. Whether you've filled the educational prescription that you requested when this patient was admitted (in order to better understand the patient's pathophysiology, clinical findings, diagnosis, prognosis, therapy, prevention of recurrence, quality of care or other important issue in order to become a better clinician). If so:
17. How you found the relevant evidence.
18. What you found. The clinical bottom line derived from that evidence.
19. Your critical appraisal of that evidence for its VALIDITY and APPLICABILITY.
20. How that critically appraised evidence will alter your care of that (or the next similar) patient. If not, when you are going to fill it.

---

* That is, a patient already known to the service.

Evidence-based Medicine

185

186

187

The sorts of words you might use:

A. Mr/Mrs/Ms/Prof/PC 11111 is a 22222 year-old 33333 44444 who was admitted on 55555 with the chief complaint of 66666.

B. They have 77777 Active Problems.

C. The first active problem is _____
It is characterized by 88888 and 99999 and we _____ which revealed 10-10-10-10.
We decided that the cause for this problem was 11-11-11-11 and we started 12-12-12-12, to which he/she responded with 13-13-13-13. We plan to 14-14-14-14.

D. The second/third/fourth active problem is _____ (repeat 8-14)

E. At the time of her/his admission, I didn't understand _____ as well as I'd like to and I requested an educational Rx to answer the question: _____

I found the relevant evidence by 17-17-17-17 and its clinical bottom line is 18-18-18-18. I believe that this bottom line is/is not valid because 19a-19a-19a-19a and I believe that it is/is not applicable because 19b-19b-19b-19b. I therefore plan to manage this and future, similar patients by 20-20-20-20.

Small groups and 'academic half-days'

Quite often, learners from different clinical teams gather at regularly scheduled educational sessions to receive general instruction in the evaluation and management of patients. The numbers of learners at these sessions can range from a handfull to a hall-full and running them on a 'set-piece' lecture format can tax the ability of the teachers to stay enthused and the ability of the learners to stay awake. An alternative approach builds on the self-directed, problem-based EBM learning orientation and runs as follows:

1. Learners are asked to identify clinical problems for which they are uncertain about the best way to diagnose or manage affected patients (stating their uncertainties in the form of clinical questions, as in Chapter 1, specifying the patient, the intervention and the outcome of interest to them). Training programs employing this approach report a distinct

pattern in the problems that learners identify. Early on, post-graduates identify medical emergencies in which they are unsure of their skills at diagnosing and managing life-threatening situations. Many programs anticipate these concerns and have basic and advanced cardiac and/or trauma support training at the ready.

2. Once the foregoing concerns are addressed, postgraduates identify a wide array of management problems in which they are not sure how to treat patients with specific disorders, followed by clinical problems in diagnosis, prognosis and etiology (especially for iatrogenic disorders). Occasionally, interest is expressed in a locally occurring quality of care study or audit, in their own continuing education, and in health economics. When several learners identify the same clinical situation,* it joins the schedule for a future session and the following processes occur:

• Acting in rotation, one or more of the learners takes on the task of searching the clinical literature for valid, relevant systematic reviews or primary articles on the clinical problem. Along the way, with help from librarians as needed, they develop and hone their skills in searching for the best evidence.

• With faculty guidance, they pick the one or two articles of highest validity and relevance and these, are copied and distributed to everyone to be studied in advance of the session.

• At that session, and again with faculty guidance as needed, they lead the discussion of the validity and potential usefulness of the evidence presented in the paper. Presenters often aid the discussion by introducing CATs or other summaries and displays of the most relevant evidence. This critical appraisal is integrated with discussions of the related pathophysiology and clinical skills, with the final objective of generating a common, evidence-based approach to the clinical

---

* Part of an initial session can be devoted to reaching consensus on priority clinical problems and such discussions can be repeated as current topics are exhausted and new topics arise.

problem. In some cases, the learners may want to work with senior clinicians to generate and circulate their own guidelines for future use.

Over the years, teachers of EBM have discovered lots of ways *not* to teach effectively and several ways that seem to work. We have summarized them in the form of a set of teaching tips, which appear in Table 4.6.2.

Journal clubs

Journal clubs are dying or dead in many clinical centers, especially when they rely on a rota through which members are asked to summarize the latest issues of preassigned journals. When you think about it, that sort of journal club is run by the postman, not the clinicians or patients, and it is no wonder that it is becoming extinct. On the other hand, a few journal clubs are flourishing and a growing number of them are designed and conducted along EBM lines. They operate like the 'academic half-days' described above.

Each meeting of the journal club has three parts:

1. In one part, journal club members describe patients who exemplify clinical situations which they are uncertain how best to diagnose or manage. This discussion continues until there is consensus that a particular clinical problem,* which we'll call problem C, is worth the time and effort necessary to find its solution. Then either the member who nominated the problem or another member, based on a rota, takes responsibility for performing a search for the best evidence on problem C.

2. In a second part, the results of the evidence search on last session's problem (we'll call it problem B) are shared in the form of photocopies of the abstracts of 4–6 systematic reviews, original articles or other evidence. Club members decide which one or two pieces of evidence are worth studying and arrangements are made to get copies of the clinical problem statement and best evidence to all members well in advance of the next meeting.

---

* Stated (as in Chapter 1) in terms of a patient, an intervention (and a comparison intervention if appropriate) and an outcome.

Table 4.6.2 Some teaching tips for EBM*

Motivating learning

A. Keep the session relevant and meaningful to learners.

1. Select (or help them track down) articles that relate to patients in their care and pick 'good' articles. Types of good articles for critical appraisal purposes (in decreasing order of their liveliness potential) include those that provide:
   - ground-breaking but solid evidence at the forefront of clinical practice (especially if not yet in widespread use);
   - solid evidence that a common practice is worthless;
   - solid evidence that a common practice ought to be questioned;
   - for common or controversial practices:
     (i) a pair of articles – a bad one to trash, maybe after reading no further than the methods, plus a good one to use for decision making or,
     (ii) a bad article with high trash titres but nonetheless the best one available;
   - NOTE: solid evidence supporting current practice is an excellent place to start (so as to avoid cynicism or nihilism) but risks boring more experienced learners.

2. Start sessions with a patient's problem (real or simulated) and end sessions by coming to a conclusion about how to manage the patient

3. Save time for closure. Come to closure about both the article and the patient. Closure does not necessarily require unanimous agreement. The group may agree that the evidence is fairly solid but still not agree on individuals' decisions for the patient in the scenario.

4. If a methodological issue comes up that may sidetrack the discussion, ask the group how they want to handle it (usually it can be deferred and discussed with just the subset of learners who are interested in deeper methodology).

B. Keep the learners active.

1. Ask the learners to vote on what they would do clinically before the article is discussed. Ask them to write down their recommendations and pass in their scripts anonymously to avoid embarrassment.

2. When someone asks a question, NEVER ridicule them.

3. Turn questions back to the person asking or to the entire group: 'What does the group think?', 'Can anyone help out here?'

4. Call on people only when they feel comfortable and know it is 'OK' not to know.

5. Ask challenging (but not intimidating) open-ended questions. 'What do the authors mean by a randomized trial?' vs 'Is this a randomized trial?'

6. When bias might be present in an article, ask the group to decide if it might be important. If present, in what direction would it influence the results; i.e. would it widen or narrow a difference between groups? Do a worst case scenario analysis. Would this bias, if present and affecting all members of a group, reverse the analysis? (In other words, could this bias be a fatal flaw?)

7. When discussing diagnostic tests, go right to likelihood ratios (omit sensitivity, specificity, prevalence, etc.), go straight to the relevant 2×2 table and help the learners generate the appropriate proportions and calculations, asking them as you go along to express what the calculations mean in words. Only afterwards ask them to put names to these concepts, like sensitivity, specificity, etc.*

8. Summarize specific points during the session; check if it's OK to move on to the next topic. Stop from time to time to synthesize and summarize to show the group that there is a set of take-home messages even though full closure may not have occurred.

9. Time out: when particular problems or successes are occurring in the group dynamic, call 'time out' to divert attention to the group process rather than the clinical problem. Examine with the group what is occurring in the interaction, then call 'time in' to return to the clinical problem. Time outs can be especially useful when the teacher senses tension: call a time out, tell the group you sense tension and ask them what's going on.

C. Show your enthusiasm for critical appraisal in general and look for opportunities to compliment your specific set of learners and the work they are doing.

D. Novelty (once your team become adept at critical appraisal).

1. Use more controversial clinical topics and articles.

2. Use articles that come to different conclusions on the same topic.

3. In non-clinical situations, use role play, and scenarios. For role play, if people are reluctant, ask them to just play themselves, in the situations they find in their daily work life. Other situations to try include: courtrooms and malpractice claims, formal debates, point-counterpoint (appoint individuals to each role), hostile residents (or consultants!) on teaching rounds.

4. Introduce a 'quick challenge' for 'snap diagnosis': for an article with a fatal flaw, especially if you sense or discover that the group has not prepared in advance, start the session with: 'Quick, is there a fatal flaw in this paper and if so, what is it?'

Learning climate

A. Learners must feel comfortable identifying and addressing their limitations.

1. Be open about your own limitations and the things you don't know.

2. Use educational prescriptions (see page 33).

3. Periodically, make it a point to say that no one knows everything and that is why we are all here.

4. Encourage people to ask questions.

5. Have fun.

6. Provide feedback. Nod your head or make some reinforcing comment, especially when a correct response is given to a question or someone brings up an important issue.

B. Fight 'critical appraisal nihilism' ('No study is perfect, so what good is any of the literature?').

1. Select good articles, especially at the start.

2. Put the article into perspective in terms of what is known in the research area. This may be the first clinical trial of a new treatment.

3. Ask learners what they would look for in (or, if they are keen to do research, how they would design) a better study on this clinical issue.

4. Remind the learners that they have to use what is available in the literature for clinical decision making. Application of critical appraisal to clinical decision making is a positive process; not using critical appraisal can result in mindless adoption of faulty practices. Mindlessness is more nihilistic than questioning and seeking the right answer.

5. Separate innocent and possible problems from fatal flaws.

6. Help learners sort the literature and the clinical practice it supports into three categories: definitely useful, incompletely tested and definitely useless.

7. Remind the learners that it may be the editors' and not the authors' fault that insufficient information is provided in the published article.

---

* Like lots of the elements of EBM, these concepts are not difficult but their jargon can be mystifying, so if you can orient students to the numbers and get them to say what they mean, you can later apply the usual terms, hopefully now demystified.

* Credit for the original compilation of this list goes to Martha Gerrity and Valerie Lawrence.

C. How to handle statistics.

1. Note the difference between statistical significance and clinical importance.

2. Use the 'statistics isn't important' technique. As a tutor, don't permit the session to turn into an attempt to teach statistics. Tell group members that study methods, samples, clinical measurements, follow-up and clinical conclusions are what's important and that statistics are merely tools to help these processes. If good methods were used, the investigators probably went to the effort to use good statistics (the 'trust 'em' mode). If bad methods were used, good statistics could never rescue the study (garbage in/garbage out, the frog is a frog and not a prince).

3. Suggest the quick and dirty sample size calculations such as the inverse rule of 3 on page 107.

Group control of the session

A. Discuss the goals of the session at its beginning and check along the way on whether it's making progress, especially if the discussion seems to be getting off track.

B. Learners' agenda versus teacher's agenda.

1. Try to go with the learners' agenda as much as possible. They will not learn all there is to know about critical appraisal in one session – remember how long it took you to learn it.

2. Let the group generate their own agenda for a specific session. This may lead into uncharted territory but learning will often be increased. The unlikely outcome is that closure may not be achieved, so be on guard to reassure (and, if you can't stand the chaos, provide direction).

3. Evaluate at the end to see if all goals were accomplished and how the next session could be more productive, more learner centered, more active, more stimulating and more fun.

C. When individuals try to dominate the discussion, put down others or 'know it all', take a 'time out' and ask the group to discuss individual responsibilities to the group. This should facilitate discussion of individual responsibilities and provide energy for individuals to take more responsibility (by the loud ones lightening up and the quiet ones contributing more).

D. When individuals or the whole group clam up and won't participate (not unusual at the first session).

1. Wait the 'magic 17 seconds'. No one can stand silence for more than about 5 seconds and the tutor who knows

(and believes!) this can outwait any group or member, no matter how long it takes. Refrain from jumping in to fill the silence yourself or they'll know that they don't have to take responsibility for their learning.

2. Take a 'time out' and ask the group members to discuss individual responsibilities to the group in terms of participation.

3. A possible script of questions to get a clinical problem + clinical article session going:

- How should we manage this clinical problem?
- What was there about the clinical article that supports that clinical decision (if unanimous) or those different decisions (if group members disagree on management)? (At this point it often becomes clear that some, and maybe all, group members haven't read the article). Does anybody need time to scan the article? (If so, you may want to give them 5 minutes to see what they can glean from it.) Alternatively, you could ask them to identify the features of an article that would be most helpful to them, then assign paragraphs of the methods section to pairs of learners and have them report back to the group on how well the article met their information needs.
- In the subsequent discussion, tease out and label the critical appraisal guides (emphasizing their generic importance rather than just how well they were met by the article).
- If the group is stalled, you could give them the guides, assigning one each to pairs of group members, have them work for a few minutes in pairs and report back to the group what they concluded and how it affects their clinical decision.
- What can we conclude and use in our clinical practice? Everyone agree?
- On which clinical issues did we achieve closure? On which not? See, lifelong learning is necessary!

4. Another question to foster discussion: The methods may be sound but are the results compelling? Concepts to bring out include statistical versus clinical significance, number needed to treat, etc.

E. Cures for the 'jumping around' or 'tangent' syndrome.

1. Remember that this syndrome is not always, or even usually, a disease. It regularly leads to long-lasting competencies in the areas under discussion, especially when the disparate elements are brought together by a skilled tutor.

2. Fill in the blank spaces on a blackboard (laid out with your mind's-eye framework of the relevant list of critical

appraisal guides) as the group comes up with and discusses the relevant issues. This will allow an unstructured discussion in which learners can generate criteria, points, etc. in any order that naturally arises, yet close with a coherent, ordered summary of the key guides and issues.

3. Check your watch frequently to see how the process is going. If a lot is being generated, don't worry about keeping a particular order or you'll risk stifling creativity and active learning.

4. Try to come up with 'segues' or transitional comments to tie what might appear to be tangential issues back into the clinical business at hand.

F. Capitalize on disagreements by asking for their bases in evidence or its critical appraisal. Where possible, reconcile them as arising from the application of different critical appraisal guides or from different interpretations of evidence related to the same guide. These reconciliations can be used to involve the rest of the group and to achieve closure on the particular issue.

G. When a learner asks a question directly to the tutor, allow the question to deflect onto another member of the tutorial, by pausing or by invitation. This can accomplish two things: (a) increase the group participation, and show them that they can teach each other, (b) buy time for you to think, in case the answer isn't immediately apparent to you but you don't want to admit that too soon!

Jargon

1. Explain a concept first, then label it with the jargon term. Better yet, get the group to explain the concept.

2. Ask learners who use jargon to explain the term to the rest of the group.

Finally

Remember that those learning to practice and teach EBM usually progress through two or three levels of expertise:

1. They become very good at sniffing out biases in articles (but don't yet know their consequences). They become highly critical and risk becoming entrenched nihilists.

2. They progress to being able to identify both the presence and direction of bias, so that they can sort out whether it's tending to produce false-positive or false-negative conclusions (and can be reassured when the latter makes a positive conclusion even more, rather than less, clinically relevant). They are ready for at least intuitive sensitivity analyses. You'd like your learners to get at least this far by the end of their training.

3. They progress further and suggest (or want to learn about) ways in which the study that produced the flawed evidence could have been designed or executed that would have prevented or overcome the bias. These learners may become interested in pursuing additional education in applied research methods and should be nurtured like other budding scientists (recognizing that their colleagues may not want to pursue these methodological discussions as part of the clinical discussions).

3. The main part of the journal club session is spent in a discussion critically appraising the evidence found in response to the clinical problem the club identified two sessions ago (we'll call it problem A) and about which it selected evidence for detailed study one session ago. The evidence is critically appraised for its validity and applicability and a decision made about whether and how it could be applied to future patients cared for by members of the journal club. This is the 'pay-off' part of the session and every effort should be made to ensure that 'closure' is reached. Ideally, a CAT is generated along the way, for discussion, revision and distribution to all the journal club members.

The actual order of these three parts of the journal club meeting could be reversed, depending on local preferences and tardiness!

Grand rounds and clinical conferences

Most hospitals hold weekly sessions in the auditorium for either their entire clinical staff or one of its departments. These sessions, which go by different names in different places, are conducted in order to discuss health issues of common interest and to try to accomplish continuing education and continuing professional development. They vary enormously in their subject matter (from molecular medicine to health reform) and in the passivity of their audience and in many hospitals patients have long since disappeared from the scene.

A common thread is the attempt to instruct the audience and transfer facts to them. Alas, as we learned back in the

Introduction, such instructional forms of CME, although they may increase knowledge, don't on average bring about either useful changes in clinical behavior or improvements in the quality of care.

Could a return to the grand round of a former era improve the situation? Building on that tradition and emphasizing some principles of EBM, these meetings could take on a different flavor and convert the audience from passive to active mode. The tactics are the following:

1. The rounds begin by focusing on a specific individual patient in the care of the presenters and the patient (whenever possible), images of the patient and undigested clinical data about the patient are presented.

2. The audience are required to assess this evidence, to generate opinions on its normalcy and diagnostic, prognostic or therapeutic implications and to report their individual opinions to the assembly by show of hands. To eliminate embarrassment and encourage participation, this reporting can be done anonymously by ticking diagnostic forms and then executing two or three exchanges among neighbors so that subsequent shows of hands are known not to represent the reporter's own opinion.* Of course, this solution is unnecessary in lecture halls equipped with anonymous, keypad voting systems.

3. A critical appraisal of the relevant evidence on the diagnostic, management or other issues raised by the case is presented in an interactive fashion, requiring the audience to offer opinions on its validity and applicability.

4. A hand-out is provided at the end of the round, summarizing both the relevant evidence and the critical appraisal guides for determining its validity and clinical applicability. In this fashion, an actively participating audience not only take stands on the appropriate evaluation and management of a real patient, but also receive a carry-away reinforcement

* It works! The author has used this approach over 100 times, with clinical audiences from five continents, and reckons that it produces participation rates of over 80%. A videotape of such a round (*Clinical Disagreement about a Patient with Dysphagia*) is available from the Centre for Evidence-Based Medicine in Oxford.

and set of guides that they can apply in other, similar situations.

Lectures (for preclinical students and clinicians of all ages and stages)

This entry may appear to be out of place! How could lectures, especially for preclinical students with no clinical skills or clinical judgment, focus in an active, interactive fashion on the care of individual patients? Well, they can, based on two realizations. First, even first year premedical students already have life experiences of a wide array of illnesses: all fear contracting AIDS, most have a relative with symptomatic coronary heart disease and many know someone with breast cancer. On the first day of school, they possess an array of personal clinical examples from which to consider the entire range of EBM topics. Second, there are unorthodox ways of employing lecture halls filled with students in ways that encourage active learning around EBM. This is perhaps best introduced by an example and the one that we will employ is a lecture to a first-year premedical class in biostatistics and epidemiology at Oxford.*

1. A clinical scenario is presented (on overheads), describing the clinical history and physical examination of a patient the speaker was called to see in an emergency room (in brief, a man who smells of alcohol and feces comes in complaining of a rapidly enlarging abdomen).

2. The students are asked to form pairs and write down the two most important facts they've been given about the patient and the two most likely explanations for his presentation. The lecturer then leaves the room for 5 minutes.

3. On return (to the sound of 60 active discussions!), the students report back their judgments and it quickly becomes apparent that there is remarkable preclinical consensus on what are considered 'clinical' issues of diagnosis.

* A videotape of this lecture (*A Stercoraceous Man with a Swollen Abdomen*) is available from the Centre for Evidence-Based Medicine in Oxford.

4. The students are then asked to identify the next most useful bit of evidence about their diagnostic explanations and the ensuing discussion around the precision and accuracy of clinical signs and symptoms introduces sensitivity, specificity, pre- and post-test probabilities, likelihood ratios and the like for later use by the faculty teaching the rest of the course.

5. Once the diagnosis and initial treatment are discussed, the issue of long-term management arises and a journal article reporting a randomized trial is distributed. Students are asked to form quartets in order to take and defend stands on whether the treatment advocated in this report should be offered to the patient. The lecturer then leaves the room for 10 minutes.

6. On return (to the roar of 30 therapeutic debates!), the students again report back their judgments and why they've decided to accept or reject the therapeutic recommendations in the published paper. The discussion introduces another host of methodological topics around descriptive and inferential statistics, statistical significance, clinically useful measures of efficacy and other topics for later use by the faculty throughout the rest of the course.

The other teachers in this course kept coming back to this patient example as they introduced the principles and methods of epidemiology and biostatistics. The students reported (in addition to enjoyment) the growing realization of the manifest relevance of understanding some epidemiological and biostatistical methodology to their goals of becoming effective clinicians.

Workshops on how to practice EBM

Although clinical learners can and do acquire the skills and knowledge for practicing EBM 'on the job' as they proceed through their careers (and this is the only site where they learn how to integrate external evidence with individual clinical expertise and apply the synthesis to patients), many learners also seek opportunities for more concentrated and focused education in its critical appraisal components. For the last 15 years, such opportunities have been provided in the form of workshops of a few hours' to a few days' duration. Originated at McMaster University in Canada, the workshop format has spread to other centers and countries and has been organized by various academic and professional groups, including a group of UK medical students who, impatient with the pace of change in undergraduate medical education, organized and ran their own 5-day workshop!* These workshops have four elements in common.

First, the learning is problem based and is typically centered around clinical scenarios describing actual patients who have been in the care of one of the faculty, accompanied by relevant research evidence (usually from the clinical literature), and calling for the learners to generate and answer questions about the clinical situation. Initially, the external evidence is provided, but later it may be the result of searches performed by the participants. By the end of the workshop, the participants will be expected to begin to pose their own questions about their own patients. An example of a clinical scenario with its citation appears in Table 4.6.3 and similar 'packages' are prepared for each of the disciplines (medicine, surgery, general practice, etc.), addressing issues in diagnosis, prognosis, therapy, systematic reviews, harm, economic analysis and quality of care.

Second, learning tends to occur in small groups of 5–10 participants with one or two tutors/facilitators who are skilled in teaching EBM and in running small groups. This provides an environment that encourages active learning and often replicates the clinical team settings in which EBM will be practiced subsequently. While carefully avoiding behavioral therapy, these groups also instruct and encourage their members in more effective and efficient team function by developing and following rules such as those that appear in Table 4.6.4. Each group meeting begins by setting an agenda for the session (including setting aside time for breaks, evaluation, future planning); agreeing on the clinical problem, the roles of group members, the educational tasks and the evidence to be appraised; getting on with it (calling 'time out' when either the process or the content is getting bogged down); evaluating this session;

* Named OCCAMS for Oxford Conference on Critical Appraisal for Medical Students and involving students from England, Scotland, Northern Ireland, Germany, Sweden and Croatia.

Table 4.6.3 A clinical scenario to initiate problem-based learning around an issue in therapy

You learn that a 54 y/o man with NIDDM (on oral hypoglycemics) whose myocardial infarction you treated 6 months ago has died suddenly at home. Wondering whether you could have done more for him, you review his notes and confirm that his was, in fact, a low-risk inferior MI with no complications whose blood sugar was elevated on admission (13 mmol/L) but settled down within 3 days.

In view of the success of 'tight control' of IDDM in preventing or postponing retinopathy and neuropathy, you wonder if a more aggressive treatment of his NIDDM might have postponed his untimely death. On the other hand, you well recall how one of your Profs back in medical school insisted that insulin was atherogenic and how you should back off insulin doses when diabetics developed angina pectoris.

So you form the clinical question: 'Among patients with NIDDM who are having MIs, does tight control of their blood sugar reduce their risk of dying?'

On your own or with help from the librarian at your local postgraduate center, you find the attached article: Malmberg K et al Randomized trial of insulin-glucose infusion followed by subcutaneous insulin treatment in diabetic patients with acute myocardial infarction (DIGAMI Study). J Am Coll Cardiol 1995; 26: 57–65.*

Read it (to possibly help you, we've included bits of a book on how to read clinical articles) and decide:
1. whether it answers your question;
2. if so, what the answer is;
whether you and your hospital colleagues should review how you are treating diabetic patients with myocardial infarctions.

* It can also be found on the disk version of *ACP Journal Club/Evidence-Based Medicine* or via MEDLINE using the terms: diabetes mellitus AND myocardial infarction AND publication type=randomized controlled trial.

Table 4.6.5 A typical schedule for a workshop on how to practice EBM

Time	Sunday	Monday	Tuesday	Wednesday	Thursday	Friday
0800		Tutors' meetings				
0900		Plenary sessions on forming questions, searching, etc.				Small groups
1000		Small groups	Small groups	Small groups	Small groups	Small groups
1100		Small groups	Small groups	Small groups	Small groups	Evaluation
1200		Lunch				Good-bye
1300		Individual study or ad hoc interest group meetings or individual searching				
1400			Tutors' meeting			
1500			Tutors' meeting			
1600		Small groups	Small groups	Small groups	Small groups	
1700		Small groups	Small groups	Small groups	Small groups	
1800		Supper				
Evening	Social	Social	Study	Social	Study	Social

Table 4.6.4 How small groups succeed in learning EBM (or anything else)

1. By taking responsibility (individually and as a group) for showing up and on time; by learning each other's names, interests and objectives; by respecting each other; by contributing to, accepting and supporting individual and group rules of behavior, including confidentiality; by contributing to, accepting and supporting both the overall objectives of the group and the detailed plans and assignments for each session; by carrying out the agreed plans and assignments, including role playing; by listening (concentrating and analyzing, rather than simply preparing your own response to what's being said) and by taking (including consolidating and summarizing).

2. By monitoring and (by using time in/time out*) reinforcing positive and correcting negative elements of both:
   • 'process', regarding educational methods (reinforcing positive contributions and teaching methods; proposing strategies for improving less effective ones) and responsibility (identifying behaviors, not motives; encouraging [e.g. with eye-contact, verbally] non-participants; quieting down [e.g. move them next to tutor] overparticipants); and
   • 'content': unclear, uncertain or incorrect facts or critical appraisal principles/ strategies/ tactics.

3. By evaluating selves, each other, the group, the session and the program with candour and respect, 'celebrating' what went well (and should be preserved) and identifying what went poorly, focusing on strategies for correcting/ improving the situation.

* Time in for the teaching/learning portions of the session, especially when using role play, time out for discussions of effective/ineffective teaching/learning methods and group/individual behavior.

and planning for the next one. Thus, the learning focuses on the five steps that form the major chapters of this book:

1. forming answerable questions;
2. searching for the best evidence (workshops usually include individual tutorials by librarians experienced in teaching searching skills);
3. critically appraising the evidence (the major focus of most workshops);

4. integrating the appraisal with individual clinical expertise and applying it in practice (this element can only be carried out when workshops are spread out over longer periods of time, with regular clinical responsibilities taking place between sessions); and
5. self-evaluation.

Given the foregoing, the selection of participants (in addition to responding to consumer demand and general interest) seeks individuals who are already receptive to EBM (skeptics make important contributions to workshops and are welcome additions to the converted) and are likely to be able to apply what they learn in their clinical practice. Most evaluations suggest that small groups made up of clinicians in the same discipline (e.g. general practice, surgery, nursing, etc.) learn best, as they can work on scenarios specific to their disciplines and more readily see how they might apply the results of their growing skills in practice. The exceptions to this rule are methodologists such as epidemiologists and biostatisticians, who are often used to functioning in disparate groups and can contribute to one of any make-up. The play of chance and small numbers (surgical specialities often are underrepresented) sometimes makes for unusual combinations of disciplines and these often require additional attention to be sure that alternative scenarios are presented to maintain relevance for all members.

Third, lots of time is set aside for small group meetings, individual study and meetings of ad hoc interest groups. Educational materials are sent out well in advance (with a reassurance that not all have to be mastered before the workshop!). A typical schedule is shown in Table 4.6.5. Tutors meet daily to report progress, to make mid-course corrections in the workshop and to identify and solve problems in group function and learning (their training occurs in the 'how to teach EBM' workshops described in Chapter 5). Plenary sessions are kept to a minimum and deal only with issues best communicated in a lecture or lecture-audience participation format (a review of EBM, how to pose answerable questions, an introduction to information searching, etc.) and a final feedback and evaluation session where participants hand in their evaluation forms and suggest improvements for future workshops.

Some workshops are held in one-day or half-day sessions, spread out over longer periods of time. Less efficient for organizers, these often merge with the journal clubs described above and provide more opportunities for integrating the critical appraisals with individual clinical expertise as the EBM skills are acquired.

Fourth, participants and organizers keep in touch after the workshops in order to continue to trade ideas on how to practice EBM, how to improve future workshops and so that some of the participants can move to the next level of not only practicing EBM but teaching it as well. These workshops will be described in Chapter 5.

Further information

Get on the WWW and browse the educational resources of the Centre for Evidence-Based Medicine in Oxford by contacting the Uniform Resource Locator: http://cebm.jr2.ox.ac.uk/

Individuals interested in attending or organizing workshops in how to practise EBM can contact either the Department of Clinical Epidemiology and Biostatistics at McMaster University (1200 Main Street West, Hamilton, Ontario, Canada L8N 3Z5) or any of the Centres for Evidence-Based Practice in the UK (for example: http://cebm.jr2.ox.ac.uk/ will get you to the Website for the Centre for Evidence-Based Medicine in Oxford).

These notes are to support a learner's manual for a structured course in learning evidence-based practice in primary care. They are deliberately brief and do not replicate material reproduced in the Learner's Manual – the two should be used in conjunction. In addition, we have not replicated material available in the textbook *Evidence-based Medicine: how to practice and teach EBM*, by D Sackett, W Richardson, W Rosenberg and R Haynes (published by Churchill-Livingstone). Several of the teaching methods that can be used in this course are described on pages 188–97 of this book, and pages from *Evidence-based Medicine*, referred to in the sessions, are reproduced in full at the back of the Learner's Manual.

The educational materials for each session include:

1   A clinical scenario based on a real patient we've seen in practice.

2   The clinical question that arose from caring for this patient.

3   The searching strategy we employed in looking for external evidence.

4   The results of that search.

5   A description of the skills-training elements of Part B of the session.

6   A blank worksheet of users' guides for critically appraising that evidence for its validity and potential clinical usefulness.

7   A completed worksheet, showing what we thought of it – the answers might not be right, but they're ours!

8   A CAT summarising the article.

Although each unit can be taught as a free-standing session, their ordering is deliberate. In our experience, learners find it easier to appraise and understand the concepts of articles dealing with therapy. Once they are confident in this area, they can move on to some of the more complex concepts associated with diagnosis, prognosis and harm. Systematic reviews usually deal with issues in therapy, but again are easier to understand if the learner has previously appraised an individual trial. The Learner's Manual is structured as a seven session course, but can be used flexibly. For example, there are two therapy examples, and each might occupy a full session.

Tutors may want to consider one exemption to our suggested ordering. Formulating 3- or 4-part questions is the fundamental building block of EBP. Particularly for a group who are not used to thinking in this way, you may want to devote the whole of the first session to practising this skill (scheduled in Session 2).

If you aren't an old hand at teaching EBM, you might want to attend one of the workshops on how to teach EBM that are held at various locations each year. These workshops include plenty of chances to develop and perfect your skills in leading sessions on the critical appraisal of articles from the clinical literature. They also explore the evidence sources that are used in this course. To find out when and where the next workshop is being held, look on our web page: *http://cebm.jr2.ox.ac.uk/*

There are several different ways to lead the discussions of the clinical scenarios and papers in these sessions:

1   We suggest that you begin all of them by being sure that the learners understand the patient's biological and clinical problem and the 3- (or 4-) part clinical question.

2   The ultimate objective is to help the learners apply the users' guides to this paper and understand them well enough to be able to apply them to subsequent papers about therapy. You can accomplish this in different ways. We give some suggestions in the tutor's notes for the therapy session – these can be equally applied in the other sessions.

3   At the end you could go over the completed worksheets and CATS, or suggest the learners do this in their own time.

4   We urge you to end each session by evaluating it with the learners, identifying ways that they, you and the readings could be improved for next time.

Other resources that we have called upon in running similar courses include:

1   Two of our local librarians – Anne Lusher and Robin Snowball – who ran the session on MEDLINE searching and have developed a teaching package for undergraduate and graduate learners. They are members of the Centre and can be contacted through us if you want additional information on how they conduct their sessions.

2   Reference to the EBM book and the cards inside it – these pages are colour-coded to match the relevant cards. *Evidence-based Medicine: how to practice and teach EBM*, by D Sackett, W Richardson, W Rosenberg and R Haynes (published by Churchill-Livingstone in 1997). You may already have another reference with which you're more familiar or find more useful.

3   For you and your learners to make optimal use of this syllabus you and they will need easy access to computers that include both CD-ROM and Internet access.

4   *Best Evidence*, a CD of eight years' worth of cumulated abstracts and other materials from *ACP Journal Club* and *Evidence-based Medicine*, two journals of critically appraised articles from an array of clinical journals covering internal medicine, general practice, obstetrics & gynaecology, paediatrics, psychiatry and surgery. This resource can be ordered from the BMJ Publishing Group (PO Box 295, London WC1H 9TE; Tel: 0171 387 4499 and ask for Subscriptions; Fax: 0171 383 6662; e-mail: bmjsubs@dial.pipex.com).

5   One of the MEDLINE searching systems (we used WinSPIRS). Members of the British Medical Association can obtain 'quick searches' and access MEDLINE (via modem or Internet) at no charge (to sign up, call the BMA Library at 0171 383 6625). Individuals with Internet access can use MEDLINE free via the Pubmed system (*http://www4. ncbi.nlm.nih.gov/pubmed/*)

6   CATMaker, a software program developed at the Centre for Evidence-based Medicine for analysing, summarising and storing critical appraisals. Now finishing field testing, it can be obtained from the Centre and the next version will be added to the website.

7   The CEBM website (*http://cebm.jr2.ox.ac.uk/*) where we keep several banks of clinically useful measures on the precision and accuracy of clinical exam and lab test results (SpPins, SnNouts, sensitivities, specificities, likelihood ratios), on the power of prognostic factors, and on therapy (NNTS, RRRs and the like).

8   For demonstrating *Best Evidence*, MEDLINE searching, the CATMaker, and the web, a tested method is to use a computer projector device that displays the contents of a computer screen onto the wall for all to see.

The scenarios and papers in this particular package have been designed for tutors and learners in general (family) practice; however, they could easily be replaced by ones more appropriate for other specialities. We have used them successfully with medical students, GPs in training and trained GPs.

We look forward to receiving feedback and suggestions for how we might improve this course.

Tim Lancaster, Dept of Primary Care, Oxford University
Sharon Straus, Centre for Evidence-based Medicine at Oxford

PART A

Critical appraisal of a clinical article about therapy
(suggested minimum time allotment: 60 minutes)

Learning objectives

1 To introduce the concept of critical appraisal and the use of critical appraisal guides and worksheets.

2 To learn how to critically appraise evidence about therapy for its validity, importance and usefulness.

3 To introduce the number needed to treat (NNT) as a clinically useful measure that can be derived from research reports.

4 To stress the application of research evidence to the individual patient.

We have included two sessions on therapy. It is a popular topic with clinicians, and the concepts are usually more familiar and easier to understand than those in the later sessions. You might like to use the two sessions sequentially. The paper on treatment of diarrhoea is a good one for practising critical appraisal, but is less well suited to understanding NNTs and the application of results to individual patients. The second paper on cardiovascular risk reduction offers a good opportunity to think about the different ways of expressing the effects of treatment (RRR, ARR, NNTs). Because there are good data on calculating absolute risk for individuals (based on the Framingham equation, and conveniently packaged in the New Zealand tables), the example is well suited to considering how the NNT varies according to the absolute risk of the individual patient. You might like to spend quite a bit of time on validity issues in the first session. Then for the cardio-vascular problem, you could cover validity very rapidly (or simply state that you consider the evidence to be valid) and focus on the results and their application.

There are several different ways to lead the discussion of these and the subsequent sessions (they are discussed in greater detail on pages 188–97 of *Evidence-based Medicine*).

1 We suggest that you begin all of them by ensuring that the learners understand the patient's biological and clinical problem and the 3- (or 4-) part clinical question.

2 The ultimate objective is to help the learners apply the users' guides to these papers and understand them well enough to apply them to subsequent papers about therapy. You can accomplish this in different ways:
   - One method is to sub-divide the group and allot each small group one task from the worksheet. For example, one group looks at the methods section and applies the study guides for assessing validity, one at the results section and interprets those, and another group considers the applicability of the evidence. This is an efficient method for rapidly appraising a paper that has not been previously read, but is less self-directed.

Continued

- At the other extreme, you could initiate a free-form discussion by asking the learners to take and defend their stands on whether they would apply the paper's conclusions to the patient, and then draw the guides out of this discussion. This approach encourages self-directed learning, but is less efficient than the tutor-directed approach and requires a group who are comfortable expressing their views.

- A third, more structured, approach is to have pre-prepared summaries (possibly on overheads) of key parts of the paper (e.g. methods, results table, study population). You can ask the group what information they would want from the paper and, when prompted, show the overheads and work through them with the group. This method can work well in limited time, and can stimulate a reticent group to participate, but is relatively tutor-directed.

- Learners often struggle with numerical concepts. Try checking their understanding of RRR, ARR and NNT at the beginning. Before having them calculate NNTs from the data in the paper, you might want to show an arithmetically simple example (e.g. when the risk of an adverse outcome is 2% in the treatment group and 4% in the control group, compared to 20% in the treatment group and 40% in the control group, you have the same relative risk but very different ARR and NNT).

3   At the end you could go over the completed worksheets and CATS – since these are published in the Learner's Manual, you may want to suggest the learners come up with their own answers before they look at ours (they may disagree with us!).

4   We urge you to end each session by evaluating it with the learners, identifying ways that they, you and the readings could be improved for next time.

PART B

Asking answerable clinical questions (suggested minimum time allotment: 45 minutes)

Learning objectives

1 **To learn why the formulation of 3–4 part questions about our patients is necessary: for identifying educational tasks that can be accomplished in limited time for focusing searches for evidence.**

2 **To learn how to generate 3–4 part answerable clinical questions from our patients.**

Asking answerable questions is discussed in detail in Chapter 1 (How to ask clinical questions you can answer) of *Evidence-based Medicine*.

The strategy we suggest you follow is aimed at illustrating the importance, strategies and tactics of formulating clinical questions, especially through paying attention to 3 (often 4) parts of the question. Since this is such a basic skill in evidence-based practice, you might wish to devote the first session to it.

One method is for you to throw out a recent clinical scenario and ask the group discuss it. Usually, the group will arrive at a point of uncertainty or disagreement about an issue in diagnosis, treatment or some other clinical aspect. You can then prod them into refining their uncertainty into a structured question.

You could then break the learners up into groups of two and ask them to discuss patients they've cared for in the previous week, and ask them to generate questions they think are important concerning their patients' therapy, diagnosis and prognosis. If a group has some experience of formulating questions, you may be able to go straight to this step.

You could then reconvene the larger group, and get some of them to volunteer their questions so that you can, as a group, review and refine them until you agree that they ought to be answerable.

Note: We urge you to keep track of these questions for use in later sessions devoted to searching for the best evidence (especially if you already know that there is good evidence about them). The feedback we've received is that your learners will be disappointed if you simply forget the products of this session and fail to use them in later searching sessions.

EBM SESSION

2

TUTOR'S GUIDE

Diagnosis
and
introduction
to the
CATMaker
software

PART

A
Critical appraisal of a clinical article about diagnosis (suggested minimum time allotment: 60 minutes)

Learning objectives

1 To learn how to critically appraise evidence about diagnosis for its validity, importance and usefulness.

2 To introduce: the concept of pre-test probability and its derivation from clinical expertise; the concepts and calculation of sensitivity and specificity; the concept and calculation of likelihood ratios; the concept and calculation (or simpler derivation from the nomogram) of post-test probability from the pre-test probability; and the likelihood ratio as a clinically useful measure that can be derived from research reports.

3 To understand the superiority of likelihood ratios over sensitivity and specificity.

4 To stress the application of research evidence about diagnosis to the individual patient.

Clinicians usually enjoy the challenge of diagnosis, and it is easy to set up a clinical scenario that involves them and allows the formulation of a 3- or 4-part question. However, the epidemiological concepts are less intuitive than those for therapy. It is usually better to start with a relatively simple example. The paper on clinical assessment of fever in children has the advantage of being brief and comprehensible while having all the data needed to understand the classification and application of a diagnostic test (in this case the 'test' is a finding from the physical examination). Its disadvantage is that the clinical scenario is less gripping than a more complex diagnostic problem. We suggest you start with this example. If you want to move on to a more challenging clinical problem, you could use a patient from your own practice and track down some evidence. Or you might like to look at another example written by Tim Lancaster and Anthony Harnden (Lancaster T and Harnden A (1998). How can we improve our diagnosis of back pain? An approach to managing diagnostic uncertainty. *In: Evidence-Based Practice in Primary Care.* Risdale L (ed). Churchill Livingstone, pp. 53–77).

We suggest you:

1 Describe the clinical scenario and work with the group to formulate the question.

2 Get the group to do a rapid critical appraisal of validity using the worksheet – the paper is short enough that they can do this quite rapidly on their own or in pairs.

Continued

PART A *Continued*

3 Work with the group to understand the results. In our experience, you will need to set aside a good chunk of time (45–60 minutes) for understanding the concepts of sensitivity, specificity, predictive value, likelihood ratios and pre- and post-test probability. Indeed, you may decide you only want to cover some of these concepts and return to the others at a later date. One possibility is to go straight to likelihood ratios, but you may find this is too much of a leap – most will have some understanding of sensitivity and specificity but many will be completely unfamiliar with likelihood ratios.

There are various ways to help understanding of the concepts. In general, it is best if the learners can work through the tables and explain the concepts to each other. However, it helps to have some pre-prepared examples that are arithmetically simple if they get stuck. As with NNTs, it is much easier to understand the concept if the numbers are absolutely straightforward. We have found it helpful to encourage the learners to discard pre-conceptions about the terms, and describe the results in their own language – most people find it easier to describe the 4-box table in terms of true and false positive and true and false negatives, than to say what they mean by sensitivity and specificity.

PART B

How to use the CATMaker (suggested minimum time allotment: 30 minutes)

Learning objective

1 To be able to use the CATMaker.

In this 'skills-training' part of the session, you can hand out copies (PC or Mac) of the CATMaker and show the learners how to use it to generate and save their own one-page 'critically appraised topic (CAT)' from an article about therapy.

The advantages of the CATMaker include its ability to calculate for them the clinically useful measures of the effects of therapy and their confidence intervals.

Obviously, in order to demonstrate it either you or a co-tutor has to know how to drive this beast, and tuition on how to run it is part of our workshop on how to teach EBM. It also would be useful to have a partially-developed 'kitten' that can be loaded into your demonstration, and you could develop one yourself on a current 'hot' topic at your institution or use the one that comes with the software. At present, this is a diabetic with hyperglycaemia at the time of a myocardial infarct, and summarises the DIGAMI randomised trial of tight control on page 41 of the Jan/Feb 1996 issue of *Evidence-based Medicine*.

To obtain copies of the CATMaker, see the CEBM web page **(http://cebm.jr2.ox.ac.uk/)**.

EBM SESSION

3

TUTOR'S GUIDE

Prognosis &
searching the
evidence-
based
journals

PART A

Critical appraisal of a clinical article about prognosis
(suggested minimum time allotment: 60 minutes)

Learning objectives

1 To learn how to critically appraise evidence about prognosis for its validity, importance and usefulness.

2 To introduce: the concept of inception cohorts and their importance in the validity of studies of prognosis and the concept (but not the tedious calculation) of precision and confidence intervals.

3 To stress the application of research evidence about prognosis to the individual patient.

Some concepts are relevant to all the sessions, and you may choose to introduce them at different points. An important area is to understand and quantify the role of chance when interpreting the results of research. In our experience, the prognosis session is a good place to consider the role of confidence intervals and P values. There is a lot of numerical work in the sessions on therapy and diagnosis, and it is usually too much to include discussion of statistical significance and precision there. Now is a good time, but remember the rule for teaching numerical concepts – have some ready made examples with easy arithmetic, so the learners can concentrate on the concepts rather than calculation.

PART B

Searching the evidence-based journals
(suggested minimum time allotment: 30 minutes)

Learning objective

1 To learn how to search the evidence-based journals of secondary publications.

Tutors will need to decide whether to start teaching clinicians how to find the best evidence as we've begun here, with the easiest sources of high-yield, high-quality evidence (but employing searching systems that incorporate 'fuzzy logic' and take away the challenge of being highly precise in specifying search terms). The alternative (preferred by some tutors of EBM) is to start at the other extreme (which we introduce in the next session) with the low-yield, variable-quality primary literature which requires much stricter specification of the clinical question and the employment of search terms drawn from methodological as well as clinical considerations. Subsequent sessions cover sources of evidence (Internet and the Cochrane Library) that call for intermediate searching skills.

Continued

Continued

Searching the electronic versions (on diskette or CD) of the evidence-based journals is so much easier (there is no need to know anything about database structures, MEDLINE, MeSH terms, and all that) and is so much more rewarding (only the 2% of articles that are methodologically sound as well as relevant get into them) that more and more of us (including our librarian colleagues) start learners off with this source rather than any of the MEDLINE systems.

Eight years of the ACPJC are already available on disk (ACP Library on Disk) and both this and *Evidence-based Medicine* are available as *Best Evidence*. Both can be ordered from the BMJ Publishing Group (PO Box 295, London WC1H 9TE; Tel: 0171 387 4499 and ask for Subscriptions; Fax: 0171 383 6662; email:bmjsubs@dial.pipex.com)

You could start by confirming that this session's article was retrievable by typing in the simple couplet: 'stroke prognosis'.

It would then be important to try using this source for finding evidence about some of the questions your learners generated last week (indeed, it would be wise to try out a few of them prior to the session so that you're sure you have some 'winners').

At the close of the session, you could encourage the learners to start searching on potential topics for their presentations in Sessions 6 and 7!

PART

A

Critical appraisal of a clinical article about harm
(suggested minimum time allotment: 60 minutes)

Learning objectives

1 To learn how to critically appraise evidence about harm for its validity, importance and usefulness.

2 To introduce the concepts (but not the tedious calculations) of some clinically useful measures of harm:
   - the NNH (the number of patients one needs to treat in order to harm one of them)
   - relative risk (RR) and odds ratio (OR).

3 To stress the application of research evidence about harm to the individual patient.

We suggest following the usual structure for this session. The learners will by now have some familiarity with the epidemiological concepts from the earlier sessions. The NNH is just a variation on the NNT, and all the principles of assessing the effect of a harmful exposure are the same as for a therapeutic intervention. The usual difference is the methodology. Whereas we demand a randomised trial to show the efficacy of therapy, for assessing harmful exposure we are often reliant on observational data. In the example we have chosen, the risk of DVT with HRT, the harmful agent is a drug, and there is now both observational and randomised evidence about this adverse effect.

In observational studies, the main issue is usually the role of bias. You may want to spend a little extra time in this session thinking about how bias may enter a case-control study. But beware nihilism! If the learner identifies a source of bias, they should be challenged not just to detect it, but to make a judgement on whether this bias is likely to be large enough to overturn the reported results.

PART

B

Searching for evidence in the primary literature
(suggested minimum time allotment: 30 minutes)

Learning objectives

1 To understand how clinicians can use the efforts of the US National Library of Medicine to classify and catalogue original articles.

2 To understand how to construct high-quality searches of the primary literature using:

   - medical subject headings (MeSH)
   - 'limiters'
   - words from the free text
   - methodological filters

Continued

PART B

3 To be introduced to other databases of primary literature.

We've never seriously considered trying to teach this skill without the collaboration of expert colleagues from the library.

We strongly encourage advance planning with local librarians, trying out searches on the questions generated by your learners in earlier sessions, so that you can show them some tangible, useful results, easily and quickly obtained, right away (rather than going in 'cold' and producing a long, slow, complicated and ultimately fruitless search that will turn them all off).

One note of caution: many librarians are used to working with researchers rather than clinicians, and thus are understandably concerned that searches get **all** the relevant citations. The needs and wants of clinicians are very different, and usually are met by **just one or a few** citations of high methodological standard and relevance. We urge you to discuss this with your librarian colleagues before the session.

Efficient EBM searching strategies developed by the research librarians in the Health Information Research Unit at McMaster (that trade off the sensitivity and specificity of your searches) are included in each pack.

Tutor's Guide

PART A

Critical appraisal of a systematic review (suggested minimum time allotment: 30 minutes)

Learning objectives

1 To learn how to critically appraise evidence from a systematic review for its validity, importance and usefulness.

2 To introduce the concept that systematic reviews are superior both to individual trials (because of greater precision and the rejection/confirmation of clinically important subgroups) and to traditional reviews (because of greater validity).

3 To stress the application of research evidence to the individual patient.

The systematic review on antibiotic treatment of cough has the advantage of dealing with a common primary care issue. Its disadvantage is that the findings are essentially of no effect, so the learners cannot practice step 3 (applying the results to individual patients). We suggest using the same structure as for the previous sessions, but concentrating in this session on steps 1 and 2.

PART B

Searching for evidence in the Cochrane Library (suggested minimum time allotment: 30 minutes)

Learning objectives

1 To learn how to look for evidence in the Cochrane Library including:
   – Cochrane Reviews
   – DARE (the Database of Abstracts of Reviews of Effectiveness) the clinical trials registry.

2 To gain information about the Cochrane Collaboration (and encouragement to join it).

In demonstrating the Cochrane Library, you might want to have done enough homework to have identified some systematic reviews that are of great relevance to your learners.

A Presentations

Depending on the number of learners who are presenting their own cases, you may find that you require just one session for these (and for the introduction to the Web). In that case, you can either shorten the course or give them one 'open' session in which they can come to you for advice and help with searching for, critically appraising or summarising their evidence. Alternatively, they might wish to practice critical appraisal of papers on other topics such as economic appraisal, decision analysis, guidelines or qualitative research.

Format of presentations
(comfortably 3 per hour)

1   In groups of 10 or less, participants will present the critical appraisals they have carried out on clinical topics of their choice.

2   Reports will state the 3-part clinical question, summarise the search in one sentence, critically appraise the best article found, and discuss how the appraisal was integrated with clinical expertise and applied on that (or a similar, subsequent) patient.

3   A total of 15 minutes will be allotted for each presentation: 10 minutes for presentation and 5 minutes for group discussion.

B Searching for evidence on the WWW (suggested minimum time allotment: 30 minutes)

Learning objectives

1   To learn how to search for evidence on the WWW.

In this part of the session, learners can be shown how to access the Web including, if you wish, the web page for the Centre for Evidence-based Medicine in Oxford (*http://cebm.jr2.ox.ac.uk/*) – here there are data banks of clinically useful measures on the precision and accuracy of clinical exam and lab test results (SpPins, SnNouts, sensitivities, specificities, likelihood ratios), on the power of prognosis factors, and on therapy (NNTs, RRRs and the like), including entries from the articles used in this syllabus, plus the CATMaker and links to several other centres and sources of evidence. The handout may help orient them to the Web.

PART A Presentations

The other half of the participants will present their patients, questions, critically appraised topics and clinical conclusion.

PART B Feedback and celebration

Objectives

1 To evaluate the course (evaluation of 'practising EBM'):
   – to improve it for the next time you give it
   – to provide feedback to the developers of this course.

2 To permit the learners to evaluate their own performance ('Am I practising EBM?').

3 To decide where you and the learners want to go from here in continuing to learn and practice EBM (e.g. the clinical rounds, academic half-days, journal clubs, etc. which are described on pages 185–206 of *Evidence-based Medicine*).

The final portion of the session (and course!) can be spent evaluating the course. The forms permit written feedback, and a discussion can be held on general issues.